Remedy Notes 2

by
John Wallace

SrP Press
2003

Remedy Notes 2

© John Wallace 2003

All rights including the moral rights of the author are reserved. No part of this publication may be reproduced, stored in a retrieval system, or transmitted in any form or by any means, electronic, mechanical, photocopying, recording, or otherwise without the prior permission of John Wallace.

Published by
SRP PRESS
11, Harescroft,
Tunbridge Wells,
Kent,
TN2 5XE

+44 (0)1892 614097
books@srppress.fsnet.co.uk

Cover design by David Copsey

ISBN   0-9534491-2-2

Acknowledgements

in the creation both of this and the previous volume – *Remedy Notes* – are due to many people for their wisdom, enthusiasm, experience and encouragement during years of training and self-development. In no particular order: Robert Davidson, Tony Hurley, Sue Josling, Myriam Shivadnikar, Rachel Roberts, Mike Bridger, Hillery Dorian, Melissa Assilem, Jeremy Sherr, David Howells and Gordon Sambridge are some of the best homœopaths on the planet – if you ever have the opportunity to be treated by them, or to listen to them in a lecture or seminar, go! Their inspirational lectures (together with many hours of study and research through other *Materia Medica*, reference texts and case notes) have given shape to these remedy pictures. There may be others whom I haven't mentioned – apologies for any unintentional omission.

Thank you also to Judi Faulkner-Pulsford for proof-reading the final copy. Special thanks also to my dear wife, Susie, whose own knowledge and encouragement has helped produce this book. And love to my children Helena, Freya and Sophia – just for being there!

John Wallace

Throughout the text the following abbreviated symbols are used:
> *means better for, improved by;*
< *means worse for*
ø *means tincture*

for Susie

Contents

Ammonium Carbonicum	11	Kali Bromatum	130
Ammonium Muriaticum	17	Kali Carbonicum	134
Anacardium Orientale	21	Kali Iodatum	140
Anhalonium	26	Kali Muriaticum	145
Benzoicum Acidum	28	Lac Caninum	147
Borax	31	Lac Defloratum	154
Bothrops	38	Lilium Tigrum	156
Bowel nosodes	40	Luna	159
Bufo	44	Lyssin	161
Cannabis Indica	48	Magnesia Carbonica	168
Cenchris Contortrix	52	Magnesium Muriaticum	171
Chelidonium	55	Manganum	175
China	57	Morgan Pure	179
Cimicifuga	62	Morgan Gaertner	183
Conium	66	Naja	186
Crotalus Cascavella	72	Natrum Sulphuricum	190
Crotalus Horridus	74	Nitricum Acidum	193
Cuprum Metallicum	77	Opium	198
Curare	82	Petroleum	202
Digitalis	85	Phosphoricum Acidum	205
Dulcamara	87	Platina	207
Dysentery Co.	90	Proteus	211
Elaps	97	Ranunculus Bulbosa	216
Fluoric Acid	99	Saccharum Officinalis	218
Folliculinum	102	Sanguinaria	222
Gaertner	108	Spigelia	224
Gunpowder	112	Sulphuricum Acidum	227
Helleborus	114	Sycotic Co	229
Heracleum Pirosella	119	Tarentula Hispania	233
Iodum	125	Veratrum Album	237
Iris Versicolor	128	Zincum	242

Introduction

Homoeopathy (in America, spelled 'homeopathy') is an eclectic discipline that nonetheless has its basis firmly in Western medicine. It is a system of treatment of disease. It also treats people who may be classified by orthodox medicine as 'well' – the constitutional basis of our existence is important to a homoeopath and requires sustenance, or reinforcement, on occasion by the administration of homoeopathic remedies to prevent, not only cure, illness.

The modern founder of homoeopathy was a German doctor, Samuel Hahnemann (1755 – 1843) although there are accounts of the use of homoeopathic principles to treat the sick in much older writings: Hippocrates (he of the 'Hippocratic Oath') in the 4th / 5th century BC considered the use of substances that treated 'like with like'.

Here is the essence of homoeopathy: it approaches the treatment of people, and of animals, by giving a sick person a substance in minute doses that, if given in larger doses to a healthy person, would bring about the symptoms that are being treated. Symptoms of interest to the homoeopath are not only physical, however: mental, emotional and spiritual dis-ease are valid indicators to a remedy, and, in a classical approach, can be of more importance in treating a sick person than the physical presentation.

Introduction

Remedies are prepared from many substances: vegetable, mineral, animal, and increasingly from 'imponderables' such as colours, or moonlight (see *Luna*). There are currently in excess of three thousand acknowledged remedies in the homoeopathic pharmacopoeia – more remedies are added each year. A remedy's picture is discovered through a process of 'proving' – Samuel Hahnemann conducted the first proving with Peruvian bark (homoeopathic China Officinalis) by giving it to himself and observing the effects he experienced (he developed malaria-like symptoms even though he was in good health). The proving process has been refined and systematised so that an effective appraisal of a substance's actions on the human system (physical, mental, emotional, spiritual) can be built up. Jeremy Sherr[1] has written in recent times probably the definitive guide to the process of conducting a Hahnemanian proving.

Remedy pictures are also sometimes discovered accidentally (through poisonings, for example) or through meditative reflection, either by individuals or in groups. The UK *Guild of Homoeopaths* was active in the conduct of meditative provings for some years from the 1970's onwards and they, along with other meditative groups, were responsible for the introduction to homoeopathy of some well-known remedies: Oak, Emerald, Rose Quartz, Sea Holly (Eryngium Maritimum), Ayahuasca, Mistletoe (Viscum Album), Sycamore Seed, Earthworm (Lumbricus Terrestris) ...

Introduction

and many others! These remedies are to be found in Madeleine Evans' insightful *materia medica* entitled Meditative Provings.[2]

The purpose of this book (as with its sister volume *Remedy Notes*) is to introduce in an accessible way both for practitioners of homoeopathy and for the general reader the key aspects of some of the most commonly used or important remedies of homoeopathic treatment. Remedy pictures are never exhaustive: they are dynamic substances, much as we are dynamic organisms, and their action on an individual may change according to that person's individual and social experience. We are constantly adding to the remedy pictures even of the substances which we use frequently in homoeopathic practice.

The *potency* of a substance may also affect its action: homoeopathic remedies are produced through a system of *dilution* and *succussion* to give them their potency. The greater a dilution, the more powerful the potency (this is the magical paradox of homoeopathy!). The decision on what potency to administer depends on factors including the general presentation of complaints, the relative importance of mental or physical symptoms, the resilience of the patient, and whether an acute illness or a constitutional picture is being dealt with.

---

[1] Sherr, Jeremy: '*The Dynamics and Methodology of Homoeopathic Provings*', Dynamis Books 1994.
[2] Evans, Madeleine: '*Meditative Provings*', The Rose Press 2000.

Introduction

Remedies are readily available in lower potencies, up to 30c; these are generally useful potencies for acute cases and so are helpful for first aid prescribing. Other prescriptions should be administered by a trained homoeopath.

This book seeks to empower both practitioners and those taking remedies through knowledge. The repertories and *materia medica* used in professional practice can be time-consuming and overwhelming in their level of detail; in this book modern references and an unorthodox but lively presentation are used to help the reader to commit to memory the major aspects of the remedy. Any references to famous persons are merely illustrative and indicate an aspect of their public *persona* only. All such references are made with the best of intentions, and no disparagement is intended.

This is a book from which to learn, to be empowered and, most of all, to enjoy!

Ammonium Carbonicum

$(NH_4)_2CO_3$ Carbonate of Ammonia

A **heart** remedy (also Lachesis, Aurum)
  Circulation, **BLOOD**

  A remedy that deals with the balance of **fluids** in the body
- Also affects the **emotional realm** –*grief*, **SHOCK**, *TRAUMA* as aetiology for heart problems

Liver, heart and kidneys are connected:

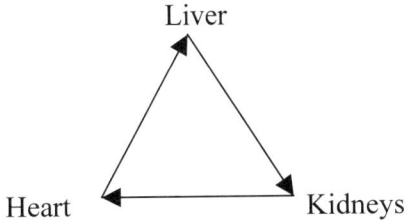

```
            Liver
            /\
           /  \
          /    \
       Heart ←→ Kidneys
```

(**Kidneys:** *also Natrum Muriaticum*)

Amm-carb patients seem OK on the surface but pathology develops later – emotional problems precede heart problems.

① *Emotional problems*
② Functional disorders
③ Tissue change
④ **Degeneration of heart**, and
⑤ Kidney disorders

Ammonium Carbonicum

"**Carb**" (*carbonicum*) = 'father',
self-worth,
VALUES,
respect,
responsibility,
dignity,
authority

"**Mur**" (*muriaticum*) = 'mother',
nurturing,
LOVE

Ammonium was *smelling salts* – smell is
**ACRID, BITTER, HARSH
Biting, caustic
RAW, ACID**

Patient emotionally is like the ammonia **smell**:

RESENTFUL,
Angry
Hate

Started out idealistic, happy
Disappointment → resentment
(with father? Establishment, society?)

BITTER
Shattered idealism

Punks

Ammonium Carbonicum

Grudge against the world
Closed people
- hold everything inside, festering

Aversion to washing
DISOBEDIENT
Children won't do what they're told
Obstinate
Possibly anarchists – *[cf. Causticum (revolutionary, idealistic)]*

Aggression is INTERNALISED and leads to **pathology:**
Sinus problems
Difficulty breathing
Weak
Low vitality

Broken down by <u>anger</u>
Can't recover from e.g. a cold

[Ammonia breaks down the mucous membranes]

CHEST AND LUNG PROBLEMS

Any discharges, e.g. leucorrhoea, are **acid, ulcerated**

Joint problems

Menstruation – exhaustion from;
- Flow is dark, excoriating

Ammonium Carbonicum

- Colic with menstruation
  (*cf. Mag Phos*)

Tendency to **OBESITY** (can be thin)
On the bigger side generally

Needs air – gasping for it

Chilly
WORSE FOR TALKING
Very **tired**, wants to lie down

Desires **high energy food –
SUGAR**
Chocolate
Easily satisfied appetite

CIRCULATORY PROBLEMS
Gets bruised, battered easily

> Blood is dark, can't clot, has a MOTTLED, PURPLISH look (*cf. Lachesis* – but *lachesis* is **warm, externalised, loquacious, passionate, jealous.**
> *Amm Carb* is **resentful, angry, not talkative, suppressive of emotions**)

Nostrils blocked
Children have runny noses, are dirty, disobedient

All mucous membranes are affected:
e.g. acrid, bleeding gums

Ammonium Carbonicum

BURNING IN INTESTINES
burning in stools
<u>Urine</u> *bloody, acid*
SKIN BURNING

** **< 3 a.m.** ** 🕒 *(also Arsenicum, the Kalis –*
syphilitic, liver and lung pathologies)

- Pneumonia at 3 a.m.
- Emphysema at 3 a.m.
- Oedema, in lungs

Listless, lethargic, low temperature

In acupuncture, <u>energy</u> goes from **LIVER** to **LUNGS** at 1 – 3 a.m.

The **LIVER** emotion is **ANGER**
(other anger remedies: Chelidonium, Nux Vomica, Lycopodium, the Magnesiums, Carduus Marianus)

The **KIDNEY** emotion is **FEAR**

The **HEART** emotions are **GRIEF, JOY**

Right sided, then left sided

Gets **AGGRAVATED, ABUSIVE**, in the evening

TALKS DURING SLEEP

Ammonium Carbonicum

Quarrelsome during **periods**

Worse for hearing people talk about them

They've let go:

'WE DON'T CARE' - SEX PISTOLS

SUMMARY:
- Idealistic *carbon* (= structure, value, worth, dignity) with *shattered ideals*
- Probably resentful attitude stemming from relationship with father, towards authority; this → rebellious, deviant behaviour/attitude
- **Closed, embittered, angry**
- Vitality diminishes, which → PATHOLOGY

Ammonium Muriaticum

NH₄Cl   Sal Ammoniac

Affects **MUCOUS MEMBRANES**
BLOOD
FEMALE ORGANS

Problems around **mother, nurturing, problems from grief** *(cf. Natrum Muriaticum)*

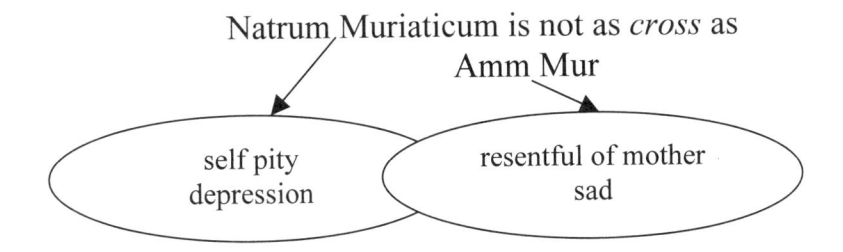

Natrum Muriaticum is not as *cross* as Amm Mur

- self pity
- depression

- resentful of mother
- sad

Amm Mur's have lost the love they wanted from the mother – she left them, died, parents have separated, worked etc. etc.

** FAT BODY, THIN LEGS **
obesity

Sluggish

** SAD BUT CAN'T WEEP **

<   A.M.   3 – 4 A.M.

Ammonium Muriaticum

> **LYING**

Will sit still: timid
Withdrawn
dignified

"Life has no love" (cf. *Natrum Carbonicum*)

Sense that they have to **protect themselves** against the savage world.

Many DELUSIONS: ***enemy under the bed***
Head surrounded by fire
A sword hanging over them

Secretions are *acid*, **acrid**, like egg white

Sinus problems
        Blocked: can't breath

> open air - don't like cold air
chilly people (*vital force is* ↓)
Right sided, then left sided

Obese, with thin legs – apple-shaped people

Ammonium Muriaticum

Most Muriaticums put on weight lower down

(Putting weight on waist and top half – indicates a problem with LIVER and GALLBLADDER *[gallbladder digests fats]*)
[Natrum Mur is the classic English pear-shape]

No **HEART** problems – *this is* Ammonium Carbonicum

Hamstrings **INFLEXIBLE**, TIGHT, **contracted**
Feels shortness of tendons

SCIATICA < sitting down
           > lying down

Resentment, with self-pity

Pain in the back and knees

Food: **desires pickles**, sour foods, **sugar**

Dislikes meat
< potatoes

Ammonium Muriaticum

[Advise patient to reduce fats, oily foods, if the presenting problem is weight distribution]
Obesity: advise less salt, possibly bread

Consider any food aggravations

Localised **pulsations**

** BOILING SENSATION IN BLOOD VESSELS AROUND BODY **

Diarrhoea and vomiting around MENSES

Burning pain, stinging in RECTUM after STOOL

Nausea

Anacardium Orientale

The Marking Nut Anacadacea
Malacca Nut
    same family as Rhus-Tox
Anacardium occidentale = **cashew nut**

Under the shell is a thick, dark, acrid juice once used for marking linen.

A **HEART** remedy

A HEART-SHAPED NUT, SURROUNDED BY BITTER, ACRID JUICE

"Ana"= "no" (*cf. Anabaptist, anaphylaxis*) : → no heart?

CRUELTY
Unfeeling
CURSING and **SWEARING**
VICIOUS
Hateful

What is underneath?

LACK OF CONFIDENCE
(Baryta Carb, Silica = lack of confidence which →
hiding away)
(Anacardium Orientale = lack of confidence covered up by cruelty, hardness)

The square peg in the round hole
in early life forced to do / be something not in their nature

Anacardium Orientale

"All my family have been doctors / lawyers, therefore I'm going to do that as well (but I'd rather be a poet)"

or they become hard:
TORTURER

** Sensation / delusion of plug in part **
∴ A BLOCKAGE IN THE ENERGY FLOW

Have never truly satisfied their heart's desire

An element of *Lycopodium* - lack of confidence covered up by bluster. *Anacardium* compensates by being tough, cruel.

Very **disciplined**

Hard on the outside, but soft in the middle

(ANNE ROBINSON)

Delusion   of mind / body SPLIT
OR HEART / MIND SPLIT
between the rational mind and emotion

HAS TWO WILLS

Anacardium Orientale

CLASH between the will, rational mind, dominating over a softer heart.

Bitterness rules the heart in the Chinese medicinal system.

Can be very unpleasant people - also lovely

Lack of bonding in motherhood

Has a **'pecking order'** approach to life

Stays in a relationship long after he/she should have left - will stick it out

AAA - Ambrogrisia, Anacardium, Arg Nit - used before examinations (embarrassment, forcing self, flapping, nerves)

They crack (like a nut) e.g. just before exams, the final challenge.

Memory gives out - struggle → split

** *They don't know what love is* **

The only thing they respect is **FORCE**

Anacardium Orientale

They control others **and** themselves

The stressed-out businessman out to prove himself, getting a stomach ulcer

** A BAND AROUND THE PARTS **
(also Platina)

** Always **better for eating**
Eating represents love - what the Anacardium lacks.

Skin symptoms are similar to Rhus Tox:
HERPETIC ERUPTIONS
VESCITIC ERUPTION

< COLD
< DAMP

hard, cold, tight, rigid - as Rhus Tox.

Useful in treating tendons

**As if there were an angel on one shoulder, a devil on the other **

Later develops a schizophrenic split

Anacardium Orientale

Sees everybody's face in the mirror except his own

Relationship difficulties between siblings: rivalry, jealousy

OBJECTS APPEAR TOO FAR OFF

Sense of smell is distorted, illusory

Peptic ulcer

Anhalonium

Peyote – cactus   Mescaline

A PSYCHOTROPIC drug – popular in the 1960's
See Carlos Castaneda: the Teachings of Don Juan

> **Insanity**
>
> **Weak HEART**

Noise and touch are seen as COLOUR
   (*cf. Cann-I*)

Heightened <u>sense</u> of colour,
taste, smell, noise, touch

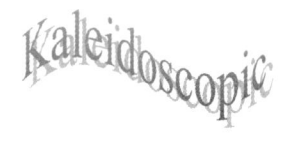

Kaleidoscopic

AUDIOVISUAL HALLUCINATIONS
SENSATION OF INCREASED PHYSICAL ABILITY

LIVING IN A FANTASY WORLD
   Losing sense of space and time

Lazy contentment

Lacking in willpower *(cf. Opium)*

Apathy
Slow reactions

Anhalonium

Sluggishness
Delusion that the body is transparent and he can see his own internal organs
Sense of INTOXICATION
Visions

MENTAL ILLNESS – SCHIZOPHRENIA

Ears: very sensitive to touch
   Sounds reverberate and make ears **PAINFUL**.

Eyes: pupils dilated *(also Cann-i)*
   Heavy-lidded
   SEES VISIONS, BRIGHT COLOURS
Natural colours seem very beautiful
Shadows seem exaggerated
Breathing   rapid and shallow

The air seems filled with perfume
   BUT ALSO

CAN LOSE SENSE OF SMELL, or
Can't differentiate between good and bad smells
Insomnia, and/or very vivid dreams
DROWSY AND DREAMY

Benzoicum Acidum

C₇H₆O₂
Benz-ac

Benzoic Acid

Acts on KIDNEYS, with symptoms extending to HEART

> ****URINE HAS A STRONG SMELL AND COLOUR****

offensive smelling, **AMMONIA**
very dark urine - ALMOST BROWN
HOT urine

Renal insufficiency

USED to combat **GOUT**

ALTERNATING SYMPTOMS:

Pains alternate between places

Pains alternate with urinary, or heart symptoms

Profuse urination alternates with scanty urination

Pains are dull, aching

Pains felt in the region of the heart
 Palpitations, < at night

Generally feels weary, feeble

Benzoicum Acidum

GOUT is worse at night. Can alternate between left and right side.

Joints become **red, swollen**.
Rheumatic symptoms

Has to draw knees up to relieve aching kidneys

ENURESIS
DRIBBLING of urine (especially in old people)
CYSTITIS

Too much uric acid

Diarrhoea is light, watery, copious
Stools are grey

Burning sensations – in kidneys, on urination, in stomach

Heat is generated from within: can feel chilly on the outside.

Can't tolerate wine

< coffee, milk

Ulcers

Mouth ulcers;
    tongue feels spongy, tender; cracked

Benzoicum Acidum

Tastes blood in the mouth

Feeling of constriction, lump, in throat; heat rising to throat

Nauseous; has no appetite in the morning

Bitter, salty taste in the mouth; needs to belch

LIVER has stitching pains

Dislikes tightness, pressure, around waist, chest, abdomen

BENZOIC ACID, BERBERIS VULGARIS, SOLIDAGO

in low potency, combined, as a kidney support and drainage combination.

Feels **WORSE** in the open air
Feels worse at night *(a syphilitic remedy)*
BETTER for heat, rest
Mainly left sided, but can alternate to right

Borax

NaBo3	Borate of Sodium

Confusion and DOUBT about identity
Emotions are very difficult to handle

Has a relation to Calc Carb

ANXIOUS, **NERVOUS**, fidgety
They sympathise with people with the same doubts and fears.

A remedy which deals with **self worth**- *father, authority (cf Calc Carb, Mag Carb) and related issues.*
    Doubts about their values
    Can't commit themselves
    Things aren't firm - no grip on themselves
Daren't say **no**

Jumpy

Fear of downward motion
    Seen a lot in children
    Child doesn't walk downstairs
    Toddlers afraid to climb down from chair
    Babies who won't go down into cot
    (cf. Gelsemium - child will cling when it's put down)
    The person putting them down is like their anchor.
Needs company, but not crowds.

Starts at slight noises -

Borax

Very, terrified, clinging.

FEAR OF THE UNKNOWN
   Anything vague frightens them

Aggravated by the sea, flying on roundabouts –
   fairground rides.

Fear of heights –*(this is a big psoric issue - but Borax is a sycotic remedy)*

Travel sickness. Anything that's not on firm ground.

CATARRHAL TYPES
   A sycotic remedy – over-production

Discharges are **thick, hot, biting**.

Affinity for MUCOUS MEMBRANES

SOFT, FLABBY types *(cf. Calc)*
Carbon types – *(cf. graphites, adamas)*

Graphite is like a tuning fork - it resonates with everything. Borax and graphite have a sensation of **cobwebs on the face**

Can also be very **emaciated** - mucous membranes can be shrivelled.

Infertility

Borax

Worse for **cold** and **damp**
Worse for **smoking**
Worse for **BEING ROCKED** *(BABY BOUNCERS!)*

Used a lot in children but also many adults

Better **11 pm**
pressure
cold weather

many stomach problems

Get irritable before stools (*downward motion*)
Can scream before passing a stool, or before urination

nappy rash - *because stools, urine very acidic*)

CRAVES SOUR THINGS - digestive tract is acidic
(cf. Medorrhinum)

Pain in stomach
Colicky children
VOMIT after drinking, with sour mucus. (*cf. Calc Carb*)

Abdomen will be **big**, **distended**, especially after a meal.

Foul-smelling stools.
Stools **burn** on passing.

Borax

*Some other sycotic remedies for children: -
Pulsatilla, Calc Carb, Medorrhinum, Thuja, Natrum
Sulphuricum*

Borax urine is **HOT, ACRID** and **FREQUENT**.

CYSTITIS – *(cf. Medorrhinum)*

Eyes: sticky, gummy, red eyelids *(Cf. Medorrhinum, Pulsatilla)*
Blepharitis

Nose: gummy, CATARRHAL, stopped up. Red.

Mouth - dry, **hot**, worse for SOUR, SALTY FOOD
ORAL THRUSH
Thrush prevents the child from nursing

Better for **alkaline**, not acidic food.
*Don't give MILK. Try soya or goat's milk.
Tomatoes, bread, dairy products, red meat are acid foods.*

Patients with skin problems often love sugar - which becomes acidic. Avoid it!

Blood group 'O' are the hunters - they need to eat meat. Wheat and dairy products upset the balance more easily for them.

Borax

Blood group 'A' are vegetarians - can assimilate wheat, dairy relatively easily.

Bowel nosodes can be appropriate - give a bowel nosode (*e.g. sycotic co, or morgan*), followed by Borax. This could sort out the digestive and bowel tract. Otherwise, give *Polybowel*. Would calm them down, make their digestive system less sensitive (also help mentally).

Female: Issues to do with *conception, pregnancy, children.*

LABOUR PAINS, EXTENDING UPWARDS. (Sepia has stitches going upwards)
Labour pains, with frequent eructations.

Pain in the opposite breast when nursing. Stitching pain.

'Borax favours easy conception'

Children stop breathing when lying down - they jump up. Used a lot with **blue babies**
Children who were stuck in the birth canal. Works well in tandem with cranial osteopathy.

Skin: dry, itchy, festers easily. Used in *Psoriasis*

Relations with other remedies:

Borax

Borax has a big relationship (**INCOMPATIBLE**) with **acetic acid** (vinegar):
Upset by wine, vinegar

Strong relationship with
Bryonia
CALC CARB
Chamomilla
Coffea
Silica (*according to Jan Scholten this is the next stage of life, when a child goes through school, puberty*).
Sulphur

Followed well by:
Arsenicum Album
Bryonia
Calc Carb
Lycopodium
Nux Vomica
Phosphorus
Silica

Antidotes:
Chamomilla
Coffea

Summary:

- **FEARFUL, NERVOUS, JUMPY**
- *Insecure*

Borax

- **Confusion about identity**
- **Easily discouraged**
- Can be happy as long as they're secure
- Clingy (but not as much as Calcarea)
- **DON'T WANT TO COMMIT THEMSELVES**
- *Lots of fear of the unknown* (cf Graphites
  - *irresolution, timidity, lack of self confidence, will cry easily from timidity. Borax is more obstinate than Graphites*)
- **Skin problems**
- **Catarrhal**
- Acidic digestive tract, → SCREAMING WHILE PASSING STOOLS
- They crave what makes them worse - **sour things.**
- Worse for *downward motion*

Bothrops

The Yellow Viper   Bothrops Lanceolatus

BOTHROPS is a virtually unproven remedy: its provings are down to poisonings.

(In common with all other snake remedies):
  Constriction, compression inside (mental, physical or emotional)
  Throat – red, dry, constricted

  'Abandoned' sense
  Independent
  self-sufficient but with an underlying sense of abandonment
      (*there is no maternal nurturing among snakes*)

Lachesis:	left-sided
Crot:	right-sided
Naja:	right-sided (slightly)
Bothrops:	right-sided

Profoundly intelligent, **CLAIRVOYANT** religious, **spiritual**, *psychic*

Vivacity – loves colours, brightness, music

DREAMS, DELUSIONS, FASCINATION WITH DEATH
Paranoid side: sense of persecution
Fear of WATER, DROWNING

Bothrops

< after sleep

#1 REMEDY FOR **THROMBOSIS **
(particularly right-sided)

BLINDNESS – tendency to day-blindness

Forgetful of words when speaking
or
Unable to speak at all: APHASIA
or
Uses **wrong words**

NECROTISING FASCIITIS (skin sloughs off in lumps)
      GANGRENE
          Necrosis
              EBOLA VIRUS
                  ANTHRAX

Thin blood that doesn't coagulate
Bloody stools

ULCERATION   -   bleeding from eyes, nose
Cerebral haemorrhages
HAEMORRHAGES generally
Vomiting **black blood**
Very SWOLLEN, PUFFED-UP LEGS with
    varicose ulcers
A remedy for *Haemophilia*

Bowel Nosodes

Bowel Nosodes are made from bowel flora.

They were developed by **Edward Bach** (*pronounced* 'Batch') around 1912. He started his career as a bacteriologist in University College Hospital, London. In 1919 he joined the London Homœopathic Hospital He ultimately discovered and researched the effect of **flower remedies** (38 Bach flower remedies are available today).

Bach examined stool cultures.
There are two types of bowel flora:
- Lactose fermenting bacteria
- Non-lactose fermenting bacteria. This is the coli-typhoid group – Bach found this had a strong connection with chronic diseases.

Bach discovered that there were nine different groups of stool cultures within the non-lactose fermenting bacteria type which were associated with chronic diseases. He sought to make a VACCINE from these bacteria; this was given initially by injection, then orally.
An auto vaccine – a bowel nosode is, strictly speaking, an isode (same tissue), not a nosode (diseased tissue).
SARCODES are made from healthy living tissue.
He called this 'auto-isopathy'.

No provings were done on bowel nosodes – their effects were noted through clinical observation.

Bowel Nosodes

Drs Paterson, Bach, Wheeler, and Dishington all worked together. Paterson categorized the nosodes into remedies. Wheeler introduced Bach to homœopathy. Bowel flora and nosodes are needed more than ever before because of the prevalence of microwaves, antibiotics, artificial hormones and because of the poor nutritional diet many people have.

They work on a biochemical level, on the principle of replacing the healthy bacteria back into the gut. When given in homœopathic potency, the non-lactose fermenting flora mutate into other groups and then disappear – along with the symptoms of the disease. During this time the stools may change, becoming loose or constipated.

Each of the nine major groups is associated with a remedy, and a disease:

    I. **MORGAN** related to SULPHUR, CARBON remedies (e.g. Sulphur, Mag Sulph, Calc Carb, Hepar Sulph). This is sub-divided into two categories:

        i. **MORGAN PURE** related to SULPHUR, and

        ii. **MORGAN GAERTNER** related to LYCOPODIUM

    II. **PROTEUS** related to CHLORINE

Bowel Nosodes

III. BACILLUS No. 7 related to BROMINE, IODINE
For patients who are exhausted (M.E.)

IV. GAERTNER related to SILICA, PHOSPHORUS, FLUORINE, MERCURIUS VIVUS

V. SYCOTIC CO. related to THUJA, MEDORRHINUM, BACILLINUM, NATRUM SULPH

VI. DYSENTERY CO. related to ARSENICUM ALBUM, ARG NIT, PULSATILLA

VII. MUTABILE related to PULSATILLA (alternating symptoms)

VIII. FAECALIS related to SEPIA

IX. BACILLUS No. 10 related to SEPIA, THUJA, NATRUM SULPH, CALC PHOS

POLYBOWEL (also known as **POLYVALENT**) is a mixture of all the bowel nosodes.

Potency: prescribe HIGH with the nosode and low for the related homœopathic remedy if mental symptoms fit. For skin problems, stay on LOW potencies.

Bowel Nosodes

> *The rule for bowel nosodes: do not change*
> (or if given in high potency repeat)
> *within 3 months*

Nosodes are given as homœopathic remedies: the practitioner looks to find the SIMILLIMUM, seeks to establish what remedy group the patient is in and identifies the nosode from this.

When do you use a bowel nosode?

- If it is a new case, and within a group, and is a clearly defined remedy, give the **remedy**. If the case relapses, give the **nosode**.

- If it is an old case, and the remedy is no longer working, give the **nosode**.

- If there are a number of equally indicated remedies, consider a **nosode** which might cover all the presenting symptoms.

Refer to the alphabetical listings for further information on the bowel nosodes

Bufo

Toad   Bufo Rana

Disposition to masturbate alone
    Cf. Agaricus – childishness
        Weak mindedness

More and more bufo types are emerging: possibly due to the increased availability of pornography. Often they are otherwise "straight" businessmen who are addicted to videos and masturbation

Weak intellectual faculty
Imbecility
Gross insensitivity

Epilepsy, convulsions *followed by unconsciousness*

   In the past, epilepsy was associated with <u>possession</u>. The secretion of the toad is an **hallucinogen** *– it takes you out of yourself into an imaginary world. Toads have variously been associated with the occult, the underworld, the* **moon***.*

PRIMITIVE
    A PRIMITIVE SEXUALITY

MORAL DEPRAVITY

      Fears of animals and strangers

Angry if misunderstood (*cf.* Ignatia)

Bufo

Can't express themselves: → *an* **EXPLOSION** *of rage – like an epileptic attack*

Idiocy
Silly tittering　　　　　　　　　　Teenagers
Talks nonsense

Dullness
Deceitful and cunning
An inclination to **bite**

MUSIC CAN BE UNBEARABLE – **the least noise distresses**

The mind remains childish – only the body grows

DOWN'S SYNDROME

May have a **TOAD-LIKE** appearance
e.g. squat, short neck, thick-set

SCHIZOID – *Bufos are afraid of their other side*

Brain-damaged, with epileptic fits

Anxious
Wrings hands

Bufo

As a poison, it acts on the circular muscle fibres: causes constriction

(Throat, anus)

Constricts the arteries

Sexually, very hyper- or hypo-active
A disposition to handle genitals and masturbate
Sexually **obsessed (and suppressed)**

Breast Cancer
Tumours and polyps of the uterus

**Septic Lymphangitis due to injuries *(sepsis with red streaks running out from the injury)*

Fear of **INFECTION**   *poor constitutional energy*

Fear in a CROWD
Fear of being **ALONE**

Fear of the NIGHT
Fear of MISFORTUNE, *as though something would happen*
Fear of DEATH

Bufo

Aversion to the sight of brilliant objects
(opposite of Stramonium) : Fear of MIRRORS – *a reflection of themselves*
(*Cf.* Stramonium, Hyoscyamus)

Dreams of business and journeys

Can have electric-like SHOCKS *felt throughout the body*

Complementary: Calc-c
Related: Baryta Carb, Graphites, Tarentula

Carbuncles
SYPHILITIC BUBOES

ANTHRAX

Sciatica

Periodicity: "Quartan fever"

Rough, dry skin
SKIN that ***CRACKS*** and ***BLEEDS*** – *from nipples, genitals, etc.*

Cannabis Indica

Hemp

An anti-sycotic remedy *(cf. Thuja, Medorrhinum)*
Problems relating back to smoking or eating cannabis

Genito-urinary tract affections:

Gonorrhœa
N.S.U. *(non-specific urethritis)*

Kidney infections
Bladder infections

Tendency to Nephritis

Burning, passing blood on urination
Inability to pass urine easily
Urine dribbles, is painful

>Urethritis
>Discharge
>**Violent, painful erections**
>*Priapism*
>
>[Agnus Castus – for someone who has been overly sexual and is now "shagged out": **impotent**]

Change of perception – time passes slowly, miles
   seem immense distances Exaggeration of the
   senses – noise, colour

Cannabis Indica

Prone to exaggeration
"everything is beautiful..." (even when it's not)

not grounded
"FLOATY" PERSONALITIES

Nothing matters

Strong fear of going MAD, of losing control

FORGETFUL – can't finish a sentence (*also Medorrhinum*)
Forgets why he entered a room, etc.

Laughing constantly, or immoderately, at frivolous things (*not through nervousness*)

Getting the giggles
Hydrogen is a grounding remedy

FEAR OF
- EVIL
  - going mad
    - the dark
      - *night*
        - **GOING TO BED**

Cannabis Indica

Very sensitive – Clairvoyant

MAY HEAR VOICES, SEE VISIONS

Delusions of grandeur (*Cf. Sulphur, Platina*)

Thinks he's **Napoleon, Jesus**

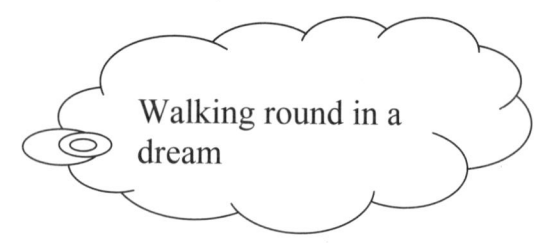

> Walking round in a dream

Physical symptoms:
- Genito-urinary tract problems
- Gonorrhœa
- **Priapism**
- **EXCESSIVE SEXUAL DESIRE**
- Pain on passing water
- *Leucorrhea in babies*

A sensation that there's something **alive** in the abdomen:
Phantom pregnancy, alien, or just an 'odd feeling'
(*Thuja, crocus, sabina, cann-i*)

Sensation of sitting on a ball (in rectum, vagina)

Threatened miscarriage

Cannabis Indica

Increased, ravenous appetite
ATTACK OF THE MUNCHIES

Sensation of **water trickling** – over head, down urethra, from heart, anus, etc.

Sensation of ***head 'opening'*** and *'closing'* (a hole in the aura from too much smoking?)

Main remedy for ill effects of other psychotropic drugs: ecstacy, LSD and similar.
    e.g. anxiety states
        slipping out of sanity
        physical effects

Loquacity
Theorising (how many angels can you fit on the head of a pin?) (*also Sulphur, Selenium*)

Not living in the here and now
Detached

Cenchris Contortrix

Copperhead Snake   Ancistrodon mokeson
Pit Viper

A remedy that very easily attacks.

IRRITATED very easily
Disturbed **sexual sphere**
VIVID DREAMS – of rape, sexual perversion, sexual torture, bestiality

SPLIT (*cf. Naja*):
Delusion of being in two different places at the same time

Delusion he will GO MAD and be taken off to an ASYLUM

Very **suspicious**, JEALOUS

Vivid, violent dreams will stay with him (her) during the day.

Very sexual, but not affectionate. **Just wants sex**.

PORNOGRAPHERS

　** Fear of pins, stings and penetration **

Alternating moods
ABSENT-MINDEDNESS
　　　with fear of going to sleep (fear they'll suffocate, have bad dreams)

Fascinated by, and terrified of, perverted sex.

Cenchris Contortrix

No **MORAL** side.

Anxiety, fear, *restlessness* (mental and physical) (*cf.* Arsenicum)

CHARISMATIC, FASCINATING, lots of **sexual energy**, desperately wanting to be appreciated.

A RIGHT-SIDED remedy (the "Right-sided Lachesis")
CHILLY

        Lachesis is left-sided, warm

Can't bear tight clothing
THROBBING of BLOOD
Difficult, empty swallowing

Aggravations from sleep
SWELLING, OEDEMA – of upper lip, of around

Aetiology: sexual abuse

eyes (*cf.* Kali carbonicum)

Cenchris Contortrix

Black leather

HAEMOPHILIA

PSYCHOPATHS

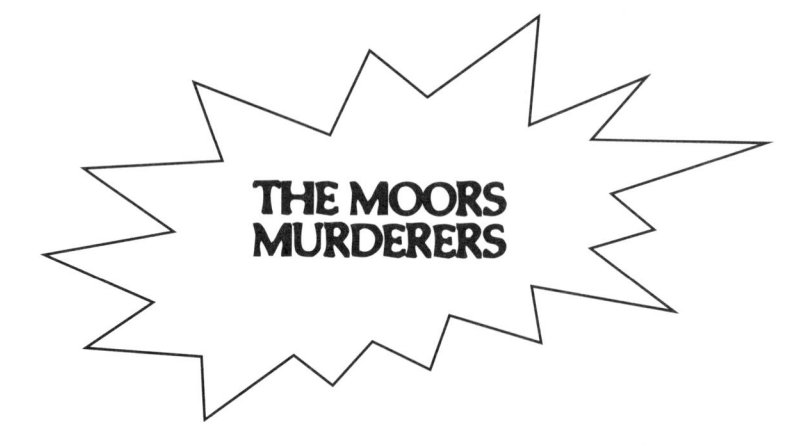

THE MOORS MURDERERS

Chelidonium

Chelidonium majus   Celandine

A **LIVER** remedy

Anger, frustration

DESIRES TO BEAT THEIR CHILDREN

Pressure, **ANGER**, frustration that comes on with someone who just wants to lash out

(Lycpodium will want to run away from their children)

Practical, matter of fact people (cf. Lycopodium, Nat Sulph)
Right-sided, left-brained

DOERS - not emotional people

Dogmatic, domineering (all liver issues)
BULLYING

HEPATITIS
Dysentery
MALARIA
ALCOHOL-INDUCED disruption of the **LIVER**

Excellent given in ø or low potency as a **LIVER SUPPORT**

Unlike Lycopodium, Chelidonium is not fearful - of authority

Chelidonium

Lethargic; **drowsy**; *awakes unrefreshed*. Wakes up repeatedly at night, and is TERRIFIED. MUST fall asleep after lunch

<   *motion*,
     cough,
     changes of weather,
     4 am and 4 pm

>   *hot food*
     PRESSURE
     EATING
     MILK
     HOT BATHS
     LYING ON ABDOMEN

China

China Officinalis   Chinchona
Quinine   Peruvian Bark

Hahnemann's first remedy

Same family as Ipecac, Coffea
An ingredient in tonic water
Relationship with Lycopodium - right sidedness,
abdominal swelling

China *constitutions* are not often seen - more often as an *acute*.

DEHYDRATION:
DEPLETED AFTER LOSS OF FLUIDS
Haemorrhages, **gastric flu**, SEVERE VOMITING

SEPSIS

Loss of fluids from any orifice
  PROFUSE SWEATING
  SUPPURATION
  DIARRHOEA
  MASTURBATION
  LACTATION
  VOMITING
  HAEMORRHAGING
A long, continuous ooze of blood: 'passive' haemorrhaging (*Phosphorus is used for an active 'gushing' of arterial blood*)

China

#1 REMEDY FOR BLOOD TRANSFUSION
give China and Phosphorus before and after

#1 MALARIA remedy

DENGUE FEVER

ARTISTIC TYPES – love beautiful colours
A sense and feel for colours

PAINTERS
Poets

Insomnia from **Fantasies** (the opposite of Natrum Sulph)
vivid thoughts, dreams

Clarity of mind at night-time

dislikes mental and physical work

Desire deep relationships
Superficial relationships don't satisfy them

A strong sense of BEAUTY

Full of ideas, plans

They believe they are unfortunate
THINK THE WORLD IS A HOSTILE PLACE

China

DELUSION of being HARASSED BY ENEMIES

irritable, *sensitive*
can't take anything said to him

Prone to **fits of temper** – want to **STAB** someone

Can be despondent, **gloomy**, **lacking a desire to live**
PERSECUTED, **paranoid**, embittered
Bitter -

Bitter flavour: **BILE**

a **LIVER** and **GALLBLADDER** remedy

Good for the **STOMACH**

Dreams of falling from a height
FEAR OF DOGS
Canine hunger or
ANOREXIA

ANAEMIA

Pale and drawn

A CHILLY remedy
Worse for cold: being cold, cold air

China

Headache: *as if the skull would burst* – throbbing, in the occiput (*cf. Belladonna, Glonoine*)

TINNITUS - ringing in the ears, with headache

FLATULENT,

- Lycopodium: distention around umbilicus / lower abdomen
- Carbo Vegetabilis: distention around pericardium / upper abdomen
- China: distention around hypogastrium / middle abdomen

Distention does not improve on burping

A good remedy for **post-operative gas**

INTERMITTENT COMPLAINTS (such as malaria)

Never been well since gastric flu

Ailments from drinking impure water (hence a good remedy for travellers to India) – *a good liver support remedy: cleanses the liver*

Hypersensitive nervous system: sensitive to **cold air**, NOISE, ODOURS

FACIAL NEURALGIA

Hiccoughs

China

Colic – *especially around 3 p.m.*

Desires TEA – drinks it all the time
Abuse of TEA

LIKES ACID FOODS AND FRUITS

Likes delicacies and dainties
Milk disagrees with them, as do oysters: gives them
GUSHING DIARRHOEA
Undigested food in stools

Oversensitive to **ODOURS**, *TOBACCO*, **COOKING SMELLS**

Cimicifuga

Black Snake-root   Actæa Racemosa

Affinity to **female organs**; mental and emotional problems; rheumatic complaints.

Acts on **NERVES** and **MUSCLES**
    LEFT SIDE of female organs

Problems in **BACK**, nape of neck, cervical **vertebrae**

Appearance: **rounded** *voluptuous*
    plumpish
        delicate   sensitive   **nervous**

(*cf. Pulsatilla: joint pains, roundish, changeable*)

Symptoms alternate beteen **mental** and **rheumatic** problems

Feels sick through **nausea, exhaustion**
[Kent: 'weakness through nursing the sick']
"Night watching" (*of a sick person*)

Symptoms are IRREGUALR, **ERRATIC**. Worse on the **LEFT**.

Very <u>CHILLY</u> (*unlike Pulsatilla*)

Cimicifuga

For problems with   MENOPAUSE
After childbirth
Epilepsy at menses
Nausea in pregnancy

Can **tone up the uterus** *(give very low potency – 1x – in the first few weeks of pregnancy)* and help to prevent **miscarriage**

Tends to have miscarriages in the 3rd month (cf. Sepia)

Use for **LABOUR** – helps dilate cervix

Problems from suppression of cervix *(cf. Lachesis)*

Lachesis is < discharge
    *Cimicifuga: **not relieved by discharge***
        *Lachesis is **warm***
            *Cimicifuga is **chilly***
    Cimicifuga is the **cold lachesis**

Both are very loquacious and jump from subject to subject (but Cimicifuga is less **witty**)

DYSMENORRHŒA continues even when menstruation starts *(cf. Mag Phos)*
Local pains are still there during periods, but the rest feels better.

Mental symptoms: **SIGHING**
                          SADNESS

Cimicifuga

50% of Cimicifuga's problems are **hormonal**
Post-natal desire to **wander** (mind and physically)
Wandering **pains**

Indecisive, not **grounded**

Nervous, fidgety, easily excited

> **Keynote:** *Fear of insanity*

Worse at menopause

"I think I'm going mad"

Depression, gloomy
Dark, heavy clouds
> *Cf. Sepia, Thuja, - walks round in circles, depressive [Princess Diana]*

Someone who goes on HRT therapy

Strong fear of RATS

Delusion she sees MICE

Fever, burning thirst, <u>not</u> anxious (∴ not aconite)

FEAR during pregnancy

Cimicifuga

Post-natally, feels as if **ENCAGED IN WIRES**; -
delusion
> *Arms and legs are bound to her body*
> **Feels restricted by the responsibility of the baby**
> Maybe feels unable to get out of a marriage (*an arranged marriage?*)

Slow delivery in childbirth

Jerking on side lain on

Conium

Hemlock
A poison

Given to Socrates to drink for "disturbing the minds of the young of Athens"

Ascending paralysis
> from the ground up: things start to paralyse and die until the brain is taken over and death ensues.

Dizziness

NAUSEA

Vomiting

"**Moving towards death**"

ARTHRITIC PARALYSIS
Hardening, indurating

Cancerous processes – hard, indurated

Cancers of the sexual organs:

> Uterine cancer
> *Prostate cancer*
> Vaginal cancer
> **Testicular cancer**
> *Breast cancer*
> Womb cancer

Conium

AILMENTS FROM SEXUAL SUPPRESSION

Ailments from enforced celibacy

Prisoners, priests, widow/ers

SLOW ONSET generally (years)

Also ailments from **EXCESSES OF LIFESTYLE**

A painless, ascending, insidious, paralysing, hardening, weakening, exhausting state

Denial, or abuse, of libido is like a movement towards death
Life-denying persons

Mind becomes dull

A gradual incapacity to focus, or memorise things (*as if the mind becomes hard, calloused*)

Children rarely need conium

Users of a lifetime of DRUGS, ALCOHOL

Also for people with an overly AUSTERE,

restrictive,

suppressive lifestyle

Conium

(Excessive overindulgence) — (Excessive denial)

↓

paralysis
induration
cancers

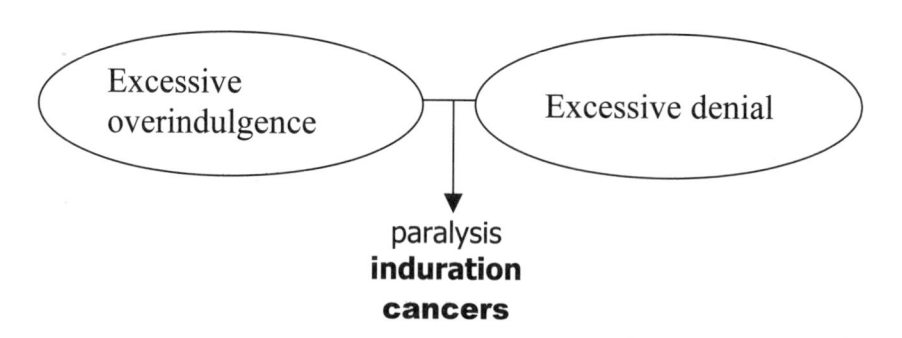

Fixed ideas
fanaticism

Superstitions

Can't pass stool, urinate, if anyone in their vicinity (cf. Natrum Muriaticum, Ambra Grisea)

Demanding
    materialistic
        OUT OF BALANCE

Conium is to Tuberculinum as Thuja is to Medorrhinum

"Delusions they threw themselves into the water
thinking themselves to be a goose"
(The goose may represent the released spirit)

Suppression of urge to be free

Conium

Basic, earthy, materialistic, sexual people

They treat people like possessions – deprivation = loss of possession
Hoarders

Sexual problems:
       Premature ejaculation
       Impotence
       Prostate problems

One of the first remedies for
       Vertigo
       Sickness
       Nausea – even when turning in bed
         > closing eyes
         < seeing moving objects

Can have a delusion of flying, but naturally rooted

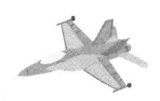

       Tabacum, Cocculus, Nux Vomica, Sepia,
                       Conium
                for **car sickness**

Stubborn
Hates to be contradicted
Premature senility
Quarrelsome
Vexatious

Conium

As soon as routine is altered

Needs people, but avoids them

Dresses inappropriately
- Dresses in finest clothes all the time
- Bag lady look
- Pancake make-up

(*inappropriate self-image*)

Buys useless things

COVETOUS, AVARICIOUS, POSSESSIVE (NOT SEETHING JEALOUSY LIKE LACHESIS)

Aetiology: shock
(may be Kali, or Calc, underneath)

Ascending ARTHRITIS
Joint problems

Animals who have been spayed and develop arthritis
HYSTERECTOMY, VASECTOMY leading to problems

**better for letting the affected part dangle **

"hang loose":

relaxation *of the part*

Conium

Loyalty

Reaction to **deprivation**

Can't pass urine – the more they strain, the more impossible they find it to go

** Aversion to light **

Cataracts

< starting to move
> confirmed movement   *Cf. Rhus Tox*

a **MENOPAUSAL** remedy

Food:
    May have been alcoholic, →
        < alcohol
        > milk

    Desires coffee (and is kick-started by it - > coffee)
    Craves SALT, SOUR THINGS, COFFEE

Dwells on the past (*cf. Natrum Muriaticum*)
Grieving (but over a lost possession)
Tormenting thoughts about **SEX**

Crotalus Cascavella

Crot-c   Brazilian Rattlesnake

Very **SOCIABLE**

Jealous

Fear of **abandonment, isolation**
Frightened of **being alone**

LOQUACITY, or IMPAIRED SPEECH

Love crowds, hustle, bustle, music

Rio Carnival!

RESTLESSNESS made worse by drinking

Gets the heebie-jeebies when under the influence of alcohol

CLAIRVOYANCE:
    sees spectres, **GHOSTS**, spirits, death
Thinks of death when alone

LAUGHING, alternating with **sadness**

Hysterical highs, deep **paranoid** lows

Lapsing into deep **apathy** –
    at worst, **suicidal** tendency

Crotalus Cascavella

Menopausal remedy (cf. Crot-h, Lachesis)

Vivacity

Forsakenness

CLAIRVOYANCE

Intolerance of clothing

Haemophilia

Crotalus Horridus

Rattlesnake

Craving for PORK (also Tuberculinum)
Craving for stimulants in general

Timid,
FEARFUL,
sad,
weepy

Crot-h people are (relatively) sociable – for snakes! *(cf. Phos)*

FEARS *cf. Phos* - thunder, lightning

Loquacious – *cf. Lachesis*
Very suspicious

Delusions of MURDER, DEATH
SMELL of DEATH
DREAMS OF DEATH

Physical characteristics:
- Very severe STREPTOCOCCAL COMPLAINTS
    - STREP THROATS
        - Haemorrhagic tendency *cf. Phos* – related to **blood**
            - **Black, dark blood**

HAEMOPHILIA

Crotalus Horridus

Eyesight DIM
          Short-sighted

< **spring, hot weather** *cf. Lachesis*
< **wine, alcohol**

Aggravated by tight clothing

Both
sympathetic, sociable
AND
suspicious, egocentric, dictatorial

Slightly less irritable than Lachesis

#1 Remedy for Coronary problems

A sense that the heart will **EXPLODE** *under the sternum*

Feeble pulse
rapid heart beat
Fluttering of heart
        "As if the heart were loose"

Alcoholic poisoning
- *Cirrhosis*
- *Toxic, septic alcohol poisoning*

Crotalus Horridus

An alcoholic in the last stages of cirrhosis

Migraines
- Vomiting of bile
- **Black**, bilious vomiting

SALLOW SKIN, YELLOW EYES
The whole body turns **YELLOW**

ALTERNATING and RECURRING pains

Fever, without perspiration: dry skin even though in a fever

Right-sided:
PARALYSIS ON THE RIGHT SIDE
Extreme sensitivity of skin on the right side

Can be HOT or COLD

A **menopausal** remedy (*cf. Lachesis, Crot-h*)

Symptoms are worse after SLEEP

Dull, heavy headaches

Vaccination – aetiology (dark, pus-filled eruptions after being vaccinated)

Cuprum metallicum

Cu　　　　　　　　　　　　　　　　　　　　　　Copper

On the 11th line of the periodic table -
A sycotic remedy

The metal of **VENUS** - same root as the word **CYPRUS** :
APHRODITE'S ISLAND (Venus island)

They are lacking that **VENUSIAN** side:
not at ease
  not sensual
    can't let go
      neurotic
        rigidly tense
      spasmodic
    contracted　　*cf. Calc Carb*

NO. 1 *convulsive and epileptic remedy*

FEEL THEY ARE UNDER ATTACK
　　　　　　Feel they need to be free
(*cf. Apis, Lachesis*)
Have completely turned off their feelings and emotions

On their guard constantly

When they finally do let go, it can be an **EXPLOSION OF RAGE**
cf Belladonna, Hyoscyamus

Cuprum metallicum

Tourette's syndrome (swearing uncontrollably)

Overbearing
Haughty
OVERPOWERING
OVERCONCERNED ABOUT THEIR SOCIAL STATUS

Selfish, misleading, *indulgent*: cxf. *Pulsatilla*

Resentful
Ruthless
Remorseless

      Grieving, with powerful emotions: yet totally closed

Deep feelings of outrage at past treatment

Exhibitionists – projecting sexuality (often inappropriately).

    LUSTFUL

    PROSTITUTES

The patron goddess of prostitutes is Aphrodite

People within SPIRITUAL GROUPS -those who want spiritual discipline, working for hours on end; zen monasteries.
Self-imposed celibacy, discipline, which ends in an explosive outburst (at worst, the epileptic attack

Cuprum metallicum

PARTY ANIMALS – life and soul of the party (*cf.* *Medorrhinum*

Full of fun, mirth, teasing, mischief;

Loves to dress up
Loves to dance
Loves **romance** and **courtship**

Practical jokers

INTUITIVE – "GUT INSTINCT"
(*Cuprum is related to the gut, lower intestine*)

Copper is a conductor of electricity: storing power, and discharging it explosively.

LOQUACIOUS

***NO. 1** remedy for burn-out, 'brain fag', mental exhaustion*

COLIC – in childhood (*also Magnesia Carbonica, Colocynthis, Dioscorea Villosa*)

A major **whooping cough** remedy
Cough with convulsions

Avoids being vaccinated

Cuprum metallicum

Used after steroid therapy, HRT (*also Nat Sulph, Thuja, Sepia*)

A female remedy –

where the "feminine" side is killed off, suppressed

> Suppression of sexuality

SUPPRESSION IS CENTRAL TO CUPRUM

> non development of conditions, suppression of conditions
> (*cf. Psorinum, Sulphur*)

Will not contribute in meetings, committees etc. (*cf. Silica*)

Meek and mild on the surface but **SEETHING** below Yielding (*cf. Zinc*) yet also **HEADSTRONG** and **EXPLOSIVE**

> Women who are normally meek but **BITE, KICK, SCRATCH, THROW THINGS** when angry
>
> *Need for social justice*
>
> A policeman's remedy - **coppers**!

Extremely **CREATIVE, ARTISTIC**
Loves COOKING – and eating: **gourmets, gourmands**

Convulsions following a **SKIN ERUPTION**

Cuprum metallicum

Lots of MOLES, **FRECKLES**, SKIN LESIONS – induced by the sun or in pregnancy

Copper is often a fair, pale person's remedy; Sepia is often a remedy for dark persons
Copper and zinc are mutually exclusive nutritionally: *do not prescribe simultaneously*

Has an AVERSION TO ORANGE

Will often wear black
(*doesn't move on; deep-seated grief*)

Arthritis - the copper bangle is often worn to relieve
although Cuprum is not generally an arthritic remedy

doesn't want to be approached

Incapable of giving, or receiving, love and affection
Natrum Muriaticum: goes into his own world
Cuprum: puts on a physical body armour:

'the metal of Venus'

CONSTIPATION
Dysmenorrhœa

Curare

Pareira brava

A poison

South American tribes tip their arrow heads with it.

Affects **MUSCLES** and **BRAIN**

PARALYSING:
The body is paralysed but the victim is conscious
(*cf. Gelsemium*)

Stephen Hawking

MOTOR NEURONE DISEASE

Used for muscle relaxation during surgical operations

Indecisive
    Unable to study
    FORGETFUL
        SLEEPY
            Mental torpor
                Depressed

Wants to be alone
Bladder, urinary complaints
kidney problems

Curare

Otitis, with a purulent discharge

CRUELTY

amoral, **VICIOUS**, unfeeling people (*cf. Anacardium, extreme Nux Vomica*)
WICKED STREAK

They **chase** people
cf. Stramonium

They have *turned away from life* - think that life is dirty, disgusting, foul
HATE PEOPLE

Hydrophobia

Kleptomania

A SYPHILITIC, destructive existence

May be fastidious about dirt, germs

Suitable in **DEBILITY VERGING ON PARALYSIS**, in old people
Consequences of *fluid loss* (*cf China*)

Irascibility
MISCHIEVOUSNESS

CHRONIC FATIGUE (*cf. Gelsemium*)

Curare

Neuralgic **headaches**, starting in forehead and radiating to neck and face (*cf. Spigelia*)

VERTIGO - sudden, with loss of feeling in legs (*cf. Conium*) Descending paralysis - from head down (Conium is ascending)

DREAMS OF FIRE

Digitalis

Foxglove

Affects **HEART** muscle circulation
Genito-urinary organs

High **blood pressure**; low **blood pressure**.

slow pulse (below 40)
Lots of OEDEMA and fluid
Cyanosis - blueness of skin

Œdema of the scrotum

Fear of DEATH during heart symptoms, or while walking

Also used allopathically. Has a cumulative effect and can cause liver problems, jaundice.

Sadness from music (*cf. Aurum*)
leading to sighing
cf. Tabacum, Lobelia (for lungs)

Despondent
ANXIOUS ABOUT THE FUTURE
Fearful
DREAMS OF FALLING

Head feels **heavy**
Deathly faint
Nausea

Digitalis

VOMITING (*which does not ameliorate nausea*)

Vertigo

One of main **arrhythmia** remedies, particularly atrial fibrillation (*Spartium for ventricular fibrillation*)

Feels as if the heart would stop beating if he moves the slightest amount (*the opposite of Gelsemium*)

One hand (or foot) cold, the other hot

Abdominal pains

Irregular breathing

Dyspnoea

Dulcamara

Bittersweet   Solanum Dulcamara

Belladonna, Stramonium, Hyoscyamus - other solanaceas
A remedy with very strong links to Calc Carb

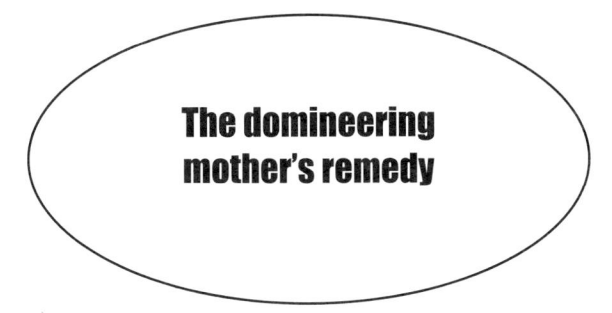

The domineering mother's remedy

The domineering matriarch

SCOLDING WITHOUT BEING ANGRY - dominates, scolds, tells off, but isn't actually angry
Strong-willed

Censorious
    Quarrelsome, without anger
HAUGHTY, ARROGANT
    Controlling
ABUSIVE, without anger

"After all you've done for me, how could you treat me like that"
"I work to the bone for you and all you can do is ...."

Dulcamara

The physical /general symptoms are important.

An AUTUMNAL remedy
< cold, damp,
Catarrh - mucous membranes are affected.

Worse on hot days followed by damp, cold nights.

Worse in the early hours of the morning, when the moisture is starting to rise

People who are constantly into hot and cold environments - e.g. a cold store

Chest infections, respiratory tract infections
An acute of the underlying calc carb tendency

Eyes - pussy, watery, mucousy: catarrhal infections that end up around the eyes (*cf. Belladonna, Stramonium, Hyoscyamus*)

A HAY FEVER remedy – profuse, watery discharge from the eyes; nose blocked, dry, or profuse watering; better indoors, or at the seaside (*cf. Nat Mur*) ; worse near cut grass.

WARTS - everywhere
Herpetic eruptions

Ailments from **exposure to the cold**:
Rheumatism, **COLD**, DIARRHOEA, asthma, spasmodic **coughs** - *like Calc Carb.*

Dulcamara

Also *cf. Rhus Tox*

Coughing for ages before phlegm is expelled

Delirium
Sees ghosts, spectres – even on waking

Confused
Finds concentration **DIFFICULT**
ANXIOUS, particularly at night
RESTLESS, AT NIGHT OR ON WAKING
Always in a hurry
Impatient
Cries with impatience

NIGHT-TIME PROBLEMS

Aversion to food; burning **thirst** for cold drinks

COLIC

Skin problems - **itching**, **PRURITUS**

** **WORSE FROM COLD AND DAMP WEATHER** **

Dysentery Co.

Dys Co. (Bach)　　　　　　　　　　A bowel nosode
　　　　　　　　　　　　　The opposite of PROTEUS

The "**HEART**" nosode.

ANTICIPATORY fears
Lots of FEARS - of high places, narrow passageways, lifts, high places, being alone, thunder, dark, etc.
Nervousness
Nerves before examinations
Inhibited, insecure types – too nervous to explode. Can't let anything out

Anxiety leads to pathology, e.g. palpitations

> Related remedies:
> Argentum Nitricum
> **Arsenicum**
> **Thuja**
> Tuberculinum

Worries about, e.g., heart disease (*c.f. Arsenicum, Kali Arsencium*)

FIXED IDEAS, OBSESSIVE
(*c.f. Thuja*)

Slow, chronic states

Shy

Dysentery Co.

Lacks confidence

"Brain fag"

FEAR OF THE FUTURE

Gets easily flustered
    Full of worries about small things

PALE, FLABBY

Physically weak

"Feels miserable from the fear that she cannot accomplish what she has to do"

Impatient
Hurried
    Restless
        Tense, unable to relax
Desire to **wander** (cf. Tuberculinum)

Depressed, gloomy, weeping

Cries easily
    Tearful before menses

Suicidal thoughts

Aggravated by **NOISE**

Vertigo
Vertigo with nausea, > lying down, < after sleep

Dysentery Co.

BLINDING HEADACHES

Frontal headaches, > fresh air
Headaches *worse before menses*
Headaches with VISIONS OF ZIG-ZAG LINES

Dandruff, dry, scaly spots

Anaemic types
Blueness of lips

Puffy eyelids
Blepharitis
styes
conjunctivitis
Flickering of eyelids
NEURALGIA

HAY FEVER

OTORRHOEA

RHINITIS

Colds all the time

Nose bleeds

Yellowness – discharges yellow; everything seems yellow with a headache

Dysentery Co.

GINGIVITIS *Bleeding gums*

ulcer on the tip of the tongue

Thyroid problems – **hyperthyroidism**

Recurrent **tonsillitis**
Dryness of throat

Constant desire to swallow;
  sensation of **LUMP IN THROAT**; choking feeling

Worse at 4 p.m.

ASTHMA – shortness of breath; worse going upstairs, on exertion. Needs to loosen collar

FIBROSITIS, neck and shoulders
Rheumatism
Spondylitis

Lumbar pains
  Back problems worse on first motion *(cf. Rhus Tox)*.
  Pains worse 9 – 10 a.m.
  Worse during warm weather
  May be useful when sulphur has failed
  Sciatic pain, especially down right leg

Pains generally better for lying down

Dysentery Co.

Indigestion, distended abdomen
FLATUS
COLITIS
Heartburn
Pains in stomach better for eating
Eructations
WATER BRASH
Indigestion from **fats, oily food**

Desires *sweets, salt, fats, milk, cheese.*
Cold food

Duodenal ulcers

Ulcers which arise out of nervous tension, especially where nerves affect the **stomach** and **heart**.
The Proteus ulcer is sudden, without warning.
Dys Co. ulcers can benefit from Lycopodium or Nux Vomica.

Scarlatina

Palpitations

Fast, irregular heart beats
Mental tension

FLUTTERING, in stomach or heart
TACHYCARDIA
Arrhythmia (*cf. Digitalis*)

Dysentery Co.

Loose stools
Yellow stools
CUTTING PAINS during stool
Itchy bottom

Arthritis: rheumatic aches and pains, stiffness, better for walking, or with exercise.

Circulatory ailments:
Raynaud's syndrome –
- Ends of fingers are swollen
- Numb hands, with dead white fingers in cold weather.
- Bluish, perspiring extremities.
- Cracked fingertips

Bruises easily
BLEEDS EASILY

Neuritis

Restless legs
"Growing pains"

INSOMNIA – waking at 2 - 3 a.m.

Skin problems: dermatitis, **ERUPTIONS**, flat **WARTS** on hands, PSORIASIS, dry, scaly eruptions.
Dry skin, ribbed NAILS, **dandruff**, *brittle hair*

Dys Co cracks heal and reveal themselves repeatedly.
Proteus cracks are deeper, with an indurated base.

Dysentery Co.

Morgan eruptions are red, hot, itchy; Dys co eruptions are scaly, crusty, purulent discharges (cf Graphites)

Chilly persons, who warm up easily.

Generally aggravate from **3 - 6 a.m**.

Elaps

The Coral Snake Elaps Corallinus

Keynotes:

** **Thick green crusts in the nose – crusty catarrhs** **

** **Very black discharges, including black ear wax** **

Elaps is the generic name for the snake family which includes the cobra (naja)

Put down, beaten, put upon - ∴ *cf. Naja*

** *Fear of falling* ** *(forward)*

FEAR of losing their position in the world, prestige, image *(cf. Lycopodium, Aurum, Veratrum Album)*

Homesick, lost

** **Fear of RAIN** ** *cf. Naja*

The Galley Slave – yanked out of his position in society, put into a galley, beaten, rained on, enslaved exposed to the elements

Right-sided paralysis
Dislikes cold things

Elaps

Cold feeling in stomach

DEPRESSED
FEAR OF BEING ALONE   **BUT**
WANTS TO BE LEFT ALONE: aversion to company
WANTS TO GO INTO THE COUNTRY
(*cf. Calc Carb*)

Angry with himself
Absorbed in his own thoughts

Playful side – **wants to frolic**
Rubric: "Desire to play in the grass"
"Snake in the grass"?

Suspicious

Fluoric Acid

HF Hydrofluoric Acid
Fl-Ac

All acids have certain qualities:

+ve:-   lively

bubbly   (like a sparkling drink)
EXTROVERT
active, FRESH
in the early stages, collapsing to

-ve: HYPERACTIVE
EXCESSIVELY HURRIED
AGGRESSIVE
and leading to
total weakness and exhaustion.

Acids want a restoration of a state of **UNITY** but they feel **alone** and **isolated**.

FLUORINE is the most reactive element in the periodic table.
Tremendous *energy*
Strong, *driving*, HEDONISTIC, vital
Incredible capacity

like a healthy Medorrhinum, Nux Vomica, Tarentula

Phenomenal **SEXUALITY**: but **AMORAL**
- *a remedy of our age*

Fluoric Acid

Obsessed with glitter, glamour, sexuality, **money** - the Glossy magazine culture

Fluorine makes teeth shiny, nice, glossy but then crumble.

SILICA often follows Fl-Ac when they go into *breakdown*

ALOPECIA (*cf. Phosphorus*) - falling hair

Neck, spinal problems (*cf. Phosphorus*)

Bones, teeth, hair, muscles, nails - all start to degenerate, **DECAY, CRUMBLE, FALL OUT.**

Fl-ac types are slightly <u>harder</u> than Phosphorus - an over-the-top edge to them: slightly more insensitive, material.

Libertarian, *LIBERTINES*

Superficiality
> never quite 'connected' with anyone
> GREED for things also REPELS them

DELUSIONS: 'BETROTHAL MUST BE BROKEN' - i.e. they'll destroy the relationship they're in (*cf. Lycopodium, but much more sexual, and no guilt*)
> They also **need** a relationship.

Fluoric Acid

Fluorine in water supply may lead to **hyperactive children** who will then crumble, with bone, teeth and spinal problems turning them into **SILICAS**.

<u>Very</u> reactive
    VENOUS CONGESTION
      Varicocities
      Early *senility*

Stands on the street, ogling women:

> **'Dirty old man'**

They've destroyed any relationship they've had
HAVE A TREMENDOUS DESIRE FOR FREEDOM

Eventually they're left alone, broken and wrecked

Finally, TOTAL INDIFFERENCE

Hot and cold aggravate (at the end: in the beginning, they can tolerate both)

A **tri-miasmatic** remedy:
    Syphilitic   Tubercular   Sycotic

May move through the remedies as follows:
    Pulsatilla → Silica → Fl-Ac (or reverse)
    Hot, → cold, → hot remedies

Folliculinum

Oestrogen

Now a very important remedy - because of the Pill, Hormone Replacement Therapy - influences which change or suppress periods.

FOLLICULINUM IS AN EXCELLENT REMEDY FOR ISSUES AROUND MENSES.

cf. Oopharinum - made from ovarian materials
Folliculinum - made from oestrogen.

Used for indiscriminate use of synthetic oestrogen.

Reconnects to earth
Similarities to Carcinosin

Typically, a woman who's lost her identity
(although can apply to men as well)

Have lost their will, identity - sexually and physically

Mental symptoms:
Anxious, hypersensitive
Easily upset
Unsure
Doesn't want to be left alone

(post-traumatic stress disorder)

Folliculinum

Confused
Indecisive
Puts on weight
Food cravings

** Keynote:

> Symptoms worse from ovulation to menstruation
> *(i.e. worse from 2 weeks before, up to period)*

    <   **heat**
    <   noise
    <   touch
    <   **resting**

    >   air

Weeps easily
History of abuse (*cf. Carcinosin*)
Mood swings
Panic attacks

All types of menstrual symptoms including **menopausal**

Ovarian cysts
           Polycystic ovaries
Cycle irregularities   **Hot flushes**
           cf. Lachesis
(Lachesis <u>drains</u> people - Foll. <u>feels</u> drained, out of control)
Fibroids
Vaginal dryness

Folliculinum

Hysterectomy *(after)*
Endometriosis
Pre-menstrual symptoms
> PMS~ PRE~MENSTRUAL SYNDROME
> *(Foll. is more pronounced than Sepia)*

Migraine
Breast pains
Diarrhoea, alternating with constipation

Food cravings - especially **sugar** and **wheat**

Recurring cystitis *(cf. Sepia)*
Abdominal bloating
Candida-like symptoms

Dysmenorrhoea
> *Painful periods*
> > Heavy bleeding
Red blood with dark clots

STRONG SEXUALITY *(also Medorrhinum)*

Aetiology: the 'morning after' pill:
> ***D.E.S.** - Diesthylstilbestrol - a man-made oestrogen used in the 1940's: Children of women given this had more vaginal cell cancers, breast cancer, abnormalities of male genitals* (low sperm count &c.). *Used to fatten animals for slaughter…*

Folliculinum

FEELS CONTROLLED BY ANOTHER

Out of sorts with her rhythms
Feels as if he's living out someone else's expectations
feels she's being fed off, emotionally or psychically
full of self-denial
a 'rescuer'
feels drained
feels like a **doormat**

Has forgotten who she is
May lose herself in her relationships
loss of identity

Used a lot in **abuse** - helps to restore the will, and empower victims

A 'grounding' remedy

> *Contra-indication:* Beware of giving Folliculinum to anyone with **skin problems**

Similar to:
  Sepia
  Pulsatilla *(but Foll. doesn't like contact: "leave me alone")*
  Carcinosin
  Lachesis
  Thyroidinum - *night sweats, hot flushes; need air*
  Natrum Muriaticum - *∴ periodicity. Natrum Muriaticum is more closed.*

Folliculinum

LUNA *(when out of tune with cycles)*
Staphysagria
Thuja
lac humanum
Proteus (a bowel nosode)
Zincum

*The POTENCY of Folliculinum is important:
   3x - 4c :   Stimulates, brings on cycle
      (∴ *good for amenorrhoea)*

    7c: most important potency.
            Regulates, balances

    9c: Suppresses - retards cycle

    30c   is commonly prescribed for hot flushes &c. Also if previously on the Pill, to detoxify (single dose only). ALSO given to men where there is a low sperm count.

Give on 10th - 14th day of cycle

Clinical indications:
   M.E. - chronic fatigue syndrome
   Raynaud's syndrome
   Palpitations
   ANGINA
   Difficulty in bonding with baby
   Children who have difficulty
       separating from parent

Folliculinum

Glandular fever

Allergies
Skin rashes
Candida

symptoms
> discharges,
< during ovulation

Excitation / depression

a first line remedy if somone wants to become pregnant, or is coming off HRT (Hormone Replacement Therapy). Can use with Mexican Yam as a supplement, and 'Progest' cream.

Gaertner
(Bach)

A Bowel nosode

Keynote: **NUTRITION**

Good for malnourished children, old people

Marked **emaciation**
Underdeveloped musculature

Fair, blue eyed, pale, thin types

Nervous people

Cold, clammy hands

Nail-biters

Excitable
Irritable
Prone to depression

Intelligent
Sensitive
FEARFUL
Conformist – eager to please (*Cf. Pulsatilla*)

Craves oatmeal (Avena Sativa)
Craves cheese, eggs, milk, sugar

Averse to bread, butter, meat, fish

Gaertner
(Bach)

Stomach aches,
Vomits everything
    COELIAC DISEASE

Inability to digest **FAT**
KETOSIS

Discharges from ears
(Give children Gaertner 30 followed by Silica 30)

Pains in back, hips

Fibrositis
Chilblains

Burning in urethra
Leucorrhoea

Slender Phosphorus types
Slim, with a pot belly; also FLABBY

    ****Projectile vomiting**** *(cf. Kali Muriaticum)*

Tend to have intolerance to **MILK**

Allergies to **TARTRAZINE, COLOURINGS**

Teenagers living on junk food
Hyperactive children

Gaertner
(Bach)

Urticarial itching
Perspiration at night

Related remedies: Phosphorus, Silica, Mercurius Vivus,
Arsenicum Album, Pulsatilla,
Chamomilla

Dysentery Co.: nervy, shy types who fidget a lot
Gaertner: mentally ill at ease – has to know everything, inspect everything. Short attention span.

Usually artistic types
Very *intelligent*
Can have a lot of *energy*

Precocious as children
"Old souls" – overdeveloped mentally (*cf. Phosphorus*) but emotionally still a child

| A remedy for WORMS |
| Used with CINA |

Gaertner follows the TUBERCULAR miasm (restless, very intelligent, bright, curious, and SYPHILITIC miasm (destructive, malignancy)

Use after RADIOTHERAPY, CHEMOTHERAPY, in CANCER.

Gaertner
(Bach)

NEVER BEEN WELL SINCE ANTIBIOTICS in children

Can get easily car sick, travel sick.

Related to Phosphorica – e.g. Natrum Phos, Kali Phos

Like Calc Carb – likes Indian food

Green vegetables, rather than red, are good for these people. Rice is OK; no dairy, foods, or bread. Oats are good. More natural foods.

NOT citrus fruits – oranges, pineapples, mangoes. Avoid sugar; aubergines; avocadoes; peanuts.

Brazil, walnuts ok (cooling foods)

Soft spoken types

They like **order, tidiness** (*cf. Arsenicum*)

Gunpowder

Made from 'black gunpowder'   nitre, sulphur & charcoal

A blood cleanser

* Blood poisoning
* **Septic states**
* Wounds that won't heal
* Ailments from drinking **bad water**
  Main remedy: Ginger (Zingiber) also China

Used to be used for gonorrhoea and syphilis.

* Infections
* **Boils**
* Abscesses
* BITES
  As an antiseptic for bites and gunshot wounds

Normally used in 3x or 6x potency - rarely used in high potency

Herpes faceonalis - herpetic eruptions on face - use **2x potency.**

Gunpowder

If scarred from herpes eruption:
Calc fluor 12x & Thios 3x T.D.S. for 1 week - 10 days

Used prophylactically to stop wound infection.

SHINGLES -esp. if vescicles nasty
VACCINATION, ill effects of
STINGS & INSECT BITES

WORMS (pref. as 2x - *low potency*)

FOOD POISONING, esp. meat (**chronic/long term**)
FOOD POISONING from watery fruits:
arsenicum

TONSILS - swollen, especially if becoming pussy
complementary remedy is **calendula**

Helleborus

The Snow Rose   Helleborus niger
Christmas Rose
Ranunculus family - also Pulsatilla, Staphysagria, Buttercup

Flowers at the **darkest** time of the year

Sense that the outside world is so terrible that they have completely cut themselves off
Virtually **catatonic**
Appalling sense of **pain** and **isolation**

Paradox that Christmas is also the time when the light is born - Yin turns to Yang
The light born out of pain and suffering

Gibson: "In the old days the philosophers used to take a draught of Helleborus before they engaged in the deepest and profoundest meditations" *i.e., it's not what you do, it's the state that you do it in.*

Major mental symptoms:

        a state of total INDIFFERENCE
        shut down
        catatonic
        NO DESIRE
        NO ACTION OF THE WILL
        the **muscles** almost **refuse to obey the will**
        the body is almost **paralysed**
    in a trance - almost needing to be shocked
back into awakening

Helleborus

AMNESIA
CATATONIA
AUTISM
Stupor
dullness

Physically, half paralysed, and jerking - epilepsy, strokes

A blank mind - *no memory*
OBJECTS APPEAR NEW
NO MEMORY OF THE PAST
SCARED, terrified, but AWED - a **mystical experience** of seeing something for the first time.

Hell, but also a potential for heaven.

Yogic mystics

Abstraction
Deficiency of ideas

Helleborus

Anything where the **memory**, **concentration** is affected

WITHDRAWN INTO THE SELF

Mind appears to have severed the link between the outside world and reality. (*Cf. Opium*)

Alzheimer's Disease

SENILE DEMENTIA

Opium, Stramonium, Helleborus - 3 remedies where there is **painlessness** where we would expect **pain**.

Possibly the most *insensitive* remedy in the Materia Medica
NUMBED

Head injury (also Arnica, Natrum Mur, Natrum Sulph)
Brain damage - to one part of the brain
    as if in a STROKE

No power of coordination - of *feeling*, *thought* or *action*.

Epilepsy

Inclination to sit

Helleborus

Old people's homes –
residents sitting lost, rocking, impassive

Long-term drug abuse
In a **VEGETABLE STATE**

After **ELECTRIC SHOCK TREATMENT**
After **chemotherapy**
After radiotherapy
After **anaesthetic** (*also Ammonium, Causticum, Carbo Veg, Camphor, Opium, Phosphorus*)

Slow, PASSIVE, painless, *withdrawn*

As if they're in a dream

Will kill themselves - if they have the will to do it

SAD _ **S**easonal **A**ffective **D**isorder

Ailments from disappointed love (*deeper than Ignatia, Natrum Mur*)

Helleborus

Suppressed SKIN ERUPTIONS

No **desire** - through **numbness**, rather than transcendence

Completely **dehydrated** *or* **œdematous**

NIGHT-BLINDNESS *(day-blindness: Bothrops)*

NO THIRST, or THIRSTY (issues about water)

Aggravated 4 - 8 p.m. *(cf. Lycopodium)*

BLOATED ABDOMEN *(cf. Lycopodium -* although Lycopodium is bloated with water, rather than wind.)

A CHILLY remedy
Dislikes cold air

A main **MENINGITIS** remedy

Aversion to **APPLES**, meat, vegetables

Heracleum Pirosella

Impure Calcium Sulphide

Made by burning Calcium (from inside of oyster shell) with flowers of sulphur (a precipitate)

Suits SCROFULOUS and LYMPHATIC constitution (often a background of tubercular adenitis (glands swollen))

Skin sensitive to touch

A deep-acting **ANTI-PSORIC** remedy

SKIN ERUPTIONS, GLANDULAR SWELLINGS.

Can be of sluggish character, with weak muscles.

Great sensitivity to all external stimuli
especially **COLD, DRY AIR** and **DRAUGHTS**

Often SWEAT easily.
Affinity for mucous membranes of respiratory tract. Produces a **CATARRHAL INFLAMMATION**.

A big **CROUP** remedy
onset very close to midnight➔ 1 - 2 am➔ 2 - 3 am

(also try ACONITE followed by HEPAR SULPH followed by SPONGIA where warm, damp air ameliorates croup)

Heracleum Pirosella

BIG TENDENCY TO SUPPURATION (PUS)

Strong symptom: **boils, abscesses**

> "the homoeopathic lance"

Can **expel** or reabsorb.
If you want to cause a 'drainage' remedy to reabsorb - give low potency
If you want everything to come out - give high potency

(*As symptoms improve support, in order, with
MERCURY➔HEPAR SULPH➔SILICA*)

Good remedy for DE-TOXING MERCURY POISONING (**dental mercury amalgam**)

** Splinter-like pains, sensation as of a FISH BONE **

All **glands** around **neck**, and **armpits** (axilla) **swollen**

Craving for SOUR or STRONG, PUNGENT things

Heracleum Pirosella

S.R.P. (*strange, rare & peculiar symptom*): "*as though a wind were blowing on a part*".

> *If patient lies persistently on one side, that side becomes intolerably painful and he has to roll over.*

A very **CHILLY** remedy.
In acutes, will get chills even moving a hand out of bed, or moving under covers.

Over-sensitivity to pain
Can become **ABUSIVE**, IRRITABLE, about pain.

Any **PRESSURE** is unbearable - gets **ANGRY**
Excessive anger in relation to condition.
Ferocious or hasty speech.

Impulses to KILL OR MURDER (with a knife)
     (*Mercury gets an impulse on seeing a knife*)

Can't bear contradiction

Tends to do everything *quickly* - eating, drinking &c.

Nothing pleases
If forced to control their anger, they may develop pathologies

The slightest stress can make them abusive

Heracleum Pirosella

> Pyromaniacs

(*cf. Calc Carb, Belladonna*: Belladonna loves to put out the fires that Heracleums start!)

STAPHYLOCOCCAL SKIN INFECTIONS

Suppuration of eyes
ULCERS of the cornea
Inflammation of the eyelids, red and painful (**blepharitis**)

Otitis media (inflammation of middle ear) with pus formation.

Tonsillitis, with great pain, *often after exposure to cold weather*

Better for warm drinks

Obstinate or chronic catarrhs, SINUS, problems with eustachian tube (*hissing* or *crackling* noises)
Catarrh is **thick** and CHEESY
Discharges smell of old catarrhs or old CHEESE

Bronchitis, with rattling cough.

Heracleum Pirosella

Asthma, worse in COLD, DRY AIR (*also aconite*)
Asthma better for dampness in air

Hoarseness, loss of voice in singers from overwork ("clergyman's throat")

Abscess at root of filled teeth
Often **scurfy**, or **eruptions** around or inside **ears**.

MASTOIDITIS (inflammation behind ear at the base of the skull)

SENSATION OF *PLUG IN PART* (eg throat)

Often crack in middle of lower lip
Excess saliva (*cf. Mercury - distinct metallic taste*)

Liver trouble
Averse to tight things around waist or abdomen

A sycotic remedy (*Sycosis - gonorrheal miasm*)
    Can develop **FIGWORTS**, CONDYLOMATA
(*for verrucas, scratch surface to roughen and apply Thuja tincture*)

BARKING coughs, like aconite

Foods: desire for ACIDS, sour things, VINEGAR, spicy foods, alcohol, PICKLES

Averse to fats

Heracleum Pirosella

Constipation
Loss of power even to expel soft stool;
even difficult to pass urine - falls vertically. (loss of muscle power)
Greasy helical on urine if left to stand.
A big **HERPES** remedy (mouth and genital)

MALE GENITAL ITCHING
Warts
Obstinate **gonorrhoea**

Worse for:
cold draft of air
    least touch
    uncovering

Better for:
    warmth
    damp

A remedy for **HEART**, kidneys, BLOOD
As a kidney organ remedy, as good as Solidago
    Best given in tincture or in low potency

Speeds the elimination of uric acid
Balances pH levels, reduces high blood pressure
Diminishes the tendency to catarrhs

A remedy for **potential stroke patients**
Add to *Arnica* and *Kali Muriaticum*
'sticky' – use when well indicated remedies get stuck

Iodum

I   Iodine
A halogen, *with Bromine, Fluorine, Chlorine*

> On the 5th line of the periodic table

Found in   the SEA
                 SALT
                 THYROID gland

*A **tubercular** remedy*

Sterilises WATER

A HOT remedy   a **reactive** remedy
Imbalances in the thyroid → HOT, HURRIED behaviour

> *Iodum is generally given for an **overfunctioning** thyroid*

THIN   EMACIATED
Eats all the time   *Cf. Natrum mur*

Burning up, overcombusting, ON FIRE

In the sea, seaweeds such as Kelp (iodine-rich) grow next to coral etc. (calcium-rich)

CALC – OPPOSITE OF IODUM

"Eating to satiety ameliorates" *(also Arsenicum, Phosphorus)*

Iodum

Fiery

Violent, murderous impulses

Generally always has a thyroid / throat problem

Overactive thyroid → **GOITRE**
EXOPHTHALMOS (bulging eyes)

Can be **OBESE**

Restless, hurried
Talkative
Needs to write lists or forgets

Thoughts are out of control, chaotic
Compulsive, neurotic behaviour, as a way of creating order

GLANDS become HARD, INDURATED *Cf.*
Tuberculinum
All glands become swollen, except mammary glands (breasts), which become shrivelled

Pounding, pulsating, throbbing throughout the body

KELP should be eaten where there is nuclear fallout (Chernobyl)

Iodum

Another Iodine-rich remedy is SPONGIA (WITH LINKS TO LUNGS, THROAT, CROUP)

Much worse for being overheated
Better for **eating to satiety**

THROAT and RESPIRATORY problems *cf. Spongia*

One of the FIRST REMEDIES IN **PANCREATIC PROBLEMS** **DIABETIC STATES**

cf. Phosphorus, Iris Versicolor

Possible aetiology: *Grief, ailments from disappointed love*

Iris Versicolor

A perennial herb, commonly found in swamps and low grounds in North America & Canada

Also known as Blue Flag. Poison Flag. Dragon Flower, Flag Lily. Snake Lily. Liver Lily. Water Flag

Acts powerfully on the **liver**

Iris root is a purgative, producing nausea, vomiting, colicky pains. Used for purifying blood.

Cathartic

Also for scrofulous complaints, and in treatment of syphilis

HEADACHES,

Eye symptoms

Digestive and **liver** problems. A useful remedy for pancreatic disturbances VOMITING, burning along digestive tract
Headache symptoms as well.
Can be **right** or **left** sided (more frequently right)
Periodicity: worse every 2 or 3 days, or weekly, 2-3 a.m., spring and autumn
MIGRAINES AFTER EATING SWEETS

Copious urination after a headache

Iris Versicolor

Visual disturbances precede headaches

Bile, *bilious headaches*
VOMITING BILE

Liver and eye symptoms are linked in Chinese medicine.

** HERPES zoster:
shingles

Shingles around the eye

Hot feet that stick out of bed at night

Worse in hot weather

Profuse, ropy saliva

Artistic, thin, delicate:(*cf. Silica*)

Charming personality

a **psoriasis** remedy

Kali Bromatum

KBr　　　　　　　　　　　Bromide of Potassium
Kali = Ash (arabic)
Pot-ash = potassium

Bromium – bromide - **suppression**
especially of *sexuality*

The *Kali* group is traditionally work-orientated, precise, duty orientated (or their opposite).

Potassium is in the 4th series of the periodic table, and the first remedy.
The "relationship" line of the periodic table.

A very *sexual* aspect to this remedy.

Delusions they are *singled out for divine vengeance*.

"Why me?"

"*Of all the people on the planet ...*"

Tremendous GUILT

Sexual excess
Puberty

The **morality** of the Kalis + the **sexuality** of the Broms = people who think they've *done something wrong* (especially about sex) and are therefore **singled out for divine intervention**

Kali Bromatum

Delusions about
> **Death**
> *Sex*
> The family

Sexual **guilt** in the family

Incest
Abuse
NYMPHOMANIA

The lid is on very tight
Religious guilt (*cf.* Thuja – but without the religious fanaticism of Thuja)

Epilepsy, convulsions

Convulsive **fits**, around **menses**
around **new moon**

Restlessness
Anxious, guilty, *fitting*

Wringing of hands

Helpless in the face of **divine vengeance** (guilt in the background)

As if Karma is dealing them one blow after another

They feel **abandoned**, by family, by God

Kali Bromatum

- feel **persecuted**
- **insulted**
- going to be POISONED
- have committed a crime

(**jump when they see a policeman**)

Dreams of being **pursued by police**

Utterly **depressed**

[Bromium is one of the **halogens** – fluorine, chlorine, bromine, iodine – all *hot* remedies)

Need to be active, busy (*cf. Rhus Tox*)

"The devil makes work for idle hands"

SUPPRESSED SEXUALITY (even → impotence)

> Kali Brom 30c: a specific remedy for teenage **ACNE**

ACNE – especially at puberty, **menses**

Croupy cough

ASTHMA; **dry cough**

The **flip side** is someone with <u>no</u> moral feeling – might turn to drink

Alcoholics

Kali Bromatum

Fear that something awful will happen
Fear that they'll get poisoned

Despair of recovery
In a **terrible state**

A **warm** remedy(because of the Bromium element)
Boiling away inside

<u>CHILDREN</u> not getting on at school
Drowsy, night terrors, *SLEEPWALKING*

Religious groups – close-knit, keeping it all in

Speedy , hot, a **<u>driven</u>** element to them.

Kali Carbonicum

K_2CO_3 Carbonate of Potassium

The **Kali** group is traditionally work-orientated, precise, duty orientated (or their opposite).

Potassium is in the 4th series of the periodic table, and the first remedy.
The "relationship" line of the periodic table.

Hard working, grafting.

Kali Carb – the typical Brit! (*cf.* Natrum Muriaticum)
    Very conservative (small 'c')
    TRADITION-ORIENTATED
    Very work-orientated
    "*back to basics*" (but with an *edge*)

Kalis tend to be OPTIMISTIC (Natrums → pessimism)

Potassium is a major ingredient of **fertilisers**: good for fruit –
    "FRUITS OF YOUR LABOURS"

If Kalis do what they have to do, "it will be all right".

Kalis need **control.** Very family-oriented people (rich in relations but with the possibility of being very limited).

Control leads to **FEAR**.
Anxiety felt in the stomach (*cf. Arsenicum, Tarentula*)

Kali Carbonicum

Typical time for Kalis is early a.m. – 2- 4 a.m. – to feel anxious in the stomach (affects diaphragm, breathing, respiration). Anxiety can be about **tasks**, family, DUTY, *guilt*.

All the Kalis are **ASTHMATIC** remedies

Anally retentive – *they hold it all in*
(∴ typical BRIT stereotypically)
- **Don't let your feelings get on top of you**
- Stiff upper lip
- Suppressed feelings

Arrogance arising out of optimism

Desires company, but treats company outrageously. Fault-finding

Physically: **big, round, tubby**
Baggy eyelids
Puffy around the eyes (because of *kidney weakness*)

Organised, principled, also
Deeply *unconventional* (but may be suppressing this) or
ECCENTRIC

A side of Kali Carb looks very much like *Calc Carb:*

Kali Carbonicum

Sweat
Backache
WEAKNESS, EXHAUSTION

Weakness in the back after sex

Not **CONTROL FREAKS** like Arsenicum, but have difficulty in letting go

Exercise a strong **mental control** over their *basic instincts*

Intellectual – not intuitive
More "left" brain than right

Entrepreneurs from the Industrial Revolution

Can be **patriarchal, benign**

Not **VIOLENT** people (but may approve of corporal punishment)

Find it difficult to **grieve**

Diseases: respiratory complaints (deep, chronic)
Pneumonia
Kidney problems
(*to do with water problems, elimination*)
kidney stones
uptight about sex
OEDEMATOUS

Kali Carbonicum

RHEUMATIC CONDITIONS
deformative arthritis
rigidity
HEART – *"as if the heart is hanging by a thread"*
(sense of weakness – just hanging on)
DIGESTION
Constipated
Stomach ulcers
Butterflies in stomach
Sweet cravers (*cf. Lycopodium, Sulphur*)
WINDY
Flatulent

(According to Kent) a difficult remedy to recognise

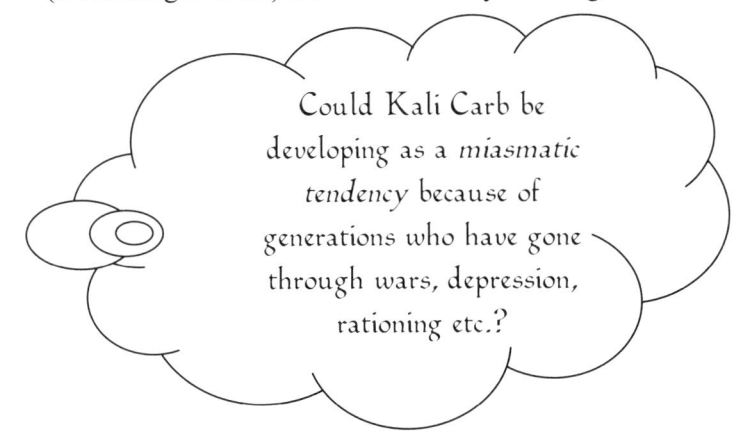

> Could Kali Carb be developing as a *miasmatic* tendency because of generations who have gone through wars, depression, rationing etc.?

Touch aggravates – have 'body armour' – especially the feet (*don't give reflexology!*)

Kali Carbonicum

Cold, *chilly* people
Draughts aggravate

"If you're not for me, you're against me"

Doesn't get involved (e.g. in a fight) – or, out of duty, wade in and stop it!

A policeman's remedy – motives are noble

BRITISH RAJ

Dry humour – Jewish humour – arising out of suffering

**Talk to themselves **

KEYNOTE: **STITCHING PAINS**
All Kali pains are sharp, **cutting**

Kali carb types are similar to Aurums – people who are hard-working, noble, guilt-ridden, but also egotistical, have to be number one, can't fail, despondent.

People who will **hoard** – security-orientated: the pension fund, insurance scheme, etc.

Very honest, **honourable**, *principled*

Kali Carb women like to wear gold and look very phosphoric. (*Lycopodium and Phosphorus types also like to wear gold; also Aurum* – *on a person who's succeeded.*) (Lyc: "I'm not insignificant – look at my gold!")

Kali Carbonicum

Summary:
1 Work, **discipline**, duty
2 Fiery, *impulsive*, *spark*
3 *A "closet eccentric"*
4 Typically "**British**"
5 Ironic, dry humour
6 Anxiety underneath it all
7 < 3 a.m.
8 STITCHING PAINS
9 **Bags over** eyes – especially upper eyelids
10 **Oedematous**
11 Weakness: sweat, backache
12 **Chilly**

Kali Iodatum

KI   Potassium Iodide

The Kali (hard work, discipline) tendency is thrown into confusion by Iodine - hyperactive

OVERACTIVE THYROID
Hot, hot blooded
Restless
BURNING
Hungry
Head full of ideas
Tubercular hyperactivity becomes **destructive**: **paranoia**, feels that he's about to be **betrayed**

Constantly busy, and needing to be free

Shows complete indifference to his children (*also Fluor Ac*)

Very **sociable**, chatty, witty

Loves fresh ideas
Loves *doing things*
Loquacity
Lively

LIFE AND SOUL OF THE PARTY

Joking
But it all ...**turns sour**:
Irresponsibility

Kali Iodatum

A SYPHILITIC remedy

GLANDULAR PROBLEMS

THROAT PROBLEMS
E.N.T. Problems

Thyroid: iodine – one of the halogens

INDEPENDENT
STRONG
Responsible
TAKES ON THE BURDEN OF THE WHOLE FAMILY, GROUP
Becomes very **IRRITABLE**
(cf. Nux Vom, but hot)
(cf. Aurum, but not dutiful, ambitious)

For problems with
    Throat – red, raw
    Nose
    Sinuses
      Swollen glands
      Headaches at the root of the nose

(Vermeulen) Watery and acrid <u>discharge</u> becoming thick, green, foul, infected
Cf.   Pulsatilla (not temperament)
       Lachesis (but no pus & infection)
       Kali Bichromicum (sinuses)

Kali Iodatum

> **TINNITUS**, in a warm-blooded person try Kali Iod 30c, single dose

A **HOT** remedy

Breasts – lumps in, or atrophy

Testicular problems

** MAJOR REMEDY FOR SCIATICA **
(*Lachesis sciatica is – unusually – right-sided*)

All Kalis have amelioration of symptoms by *moving fast*, by being in *cool, fresh air*

AVERSE TO TOUCH
Very **IRRITABLE**
QUARRELSOME
Almost *malicious*
Obstinate
Violent ANGER

Worse at NIGHT

In a completely failed state
Despair, **disgust** with everything, *insanity*

ABUSIVE
   haughty
      abrupt
         unfeeling

Kali Iodatum

What used to be a pleasure *has now become a* burden

An **ASTHMA** remedy (like other Kalis)

weakness

> For ANAEMIA try Kali Ferrocyanatum

Skin symptoms:

Deep psoriasis
Itching
Eruptions
BOILS
Very septic thread running through

> [for sepsis – think also of   Echinacea
> Pyrogen
> Stilego
> Lachesis
> Hepar sulph
> Calc sulph
> Syphilinum

HEART PALPITATIONS

Nightly BONE PAINS
FISSURES, SPLITS
Anal fissures

Kali Iodatum

DESTRUCTION OF NASAL SEPTUM
Foul-smelling **catarrh**

Can *smell* foulness - **OZOENA**

Kali Muriaticum

KCl   Potassium Chloride

A major remedy, and a tissue salt.

Confused with KALI CHLOR (Potassium Chlor<u>ate</u>)

Both have a strong tendency to ANOREXIA

Kali Chlor has delusions she must starve and refuses to eat

MOUTH ULCERS – stomatitis
Eruptions around the mouth
Aphthae (raised lumps or ulcers)
Thrush
FOUL BREATH
(*Sulphuricum Acidum*, **Borax** [Sodium Borate] – also remedies for mouth problems)

Incredibly devoted, family-orientated mothers

Constitutional tendency to:
    (KALI)   (MUR)
- **duty**   nurturing
- **work**   maternity
- **family**

Opaque, grey-white discharges
Blocked-up ear

HORROR OF **FATTY FOODS** (like their opaque, thick white mucus)
[*digestive fluid is predominantly hydrochloric acid*]

Kali Muriaticum

Physical symptoms:

#1 remedy for **GLUE EAR**

Fibrinous discharges

ASTHMA LINKED TO **DIGESTIVE PROBLEMS**
(*Muriaticum: connected with stomach
Kali : connected with lungs*)

There are very few mental symptoms for this remedy.

Cold hands and feet
CRAMPS IN LEGS

Link between **mouth, kidneys, rectum, blood**

Tendency to *Prostration*
Haemorrhaging
SALIVATION
Convulsion
COLIC, DYSENTERY

INFLAMMATION OF THE KIDNEYS with **HAEMATURIA**
(*blood in urine*)

Nephritis

Lac Caninum

Dog's milk

Of LAC CANINUM and LAC DEFLORATUM, Lac-C is the bigger remedy; a reasonably common constitutional remedy.

A very 'doggy' remedy – patients are 'doggy-like':
Sociable – like company
loyal
obedient
dutiful
protective of their young

** afraid of snakes **(also Arg Nit)

"dog-tired"

Nervous
Highly strung

Strong feelings of SELF-REPROACH
Feeling unworthy – *"disgust with self"*
Feels bad about self, mentally and physically

Lac Caninum

History of being put down a lot (suppressed)
"treated like a dog"

Given no respect – by partner, father, etc.
No self-confidence
Can be **distrusting**, **suspicious** of people's motives
Thinks people **look down on him**
Feels as though he's invisible

> GUILTY feelings – *feel they've been bad*

Strong fear of disease, especially CANCER
"Every illness is a serious disease"
"Feels she has a loathsome mass of disease" (Kent)

Born unlucky
Doubtful of their ability
Very lacking in confidence – confidence has been beaten out of them
Desire to please

Imagery associated with SNAKES "it's like a snake uncoiling .."
Strong fear of the DARK
Fear of FALLING – **especially down stairs**
DREAMS about snakes – under bed, on floor

Fear of (and possibly history of) fainting, fitting
(*also Arg Nit*)
> *Arg Nit doesn't usually have a background of abuse and desire to please*

Lac Caninum

Can become agoraphobic – gets despondent
Fear they'll lose their reason, of insanity
Forgetful
Very absent-minded

They love children

Wet-nurses:
    Might foster 20 children
        Strong desire to nurture and protect the young
        Either love, or are afraid of, dogs
        Generally dislike cats

Innocence, naivety

Some linguistic references to dogs:
    "Dog in the manger"
    Dog days (July – August)
    Dogged determination
    Dog-watch
    Dressed like a dog's dinner

Faithful, even to people who mistreat them

Stay faithful even when widowed: never remarry

Find it hard to break attachments

Lac Caninum

Nice friends to have – *they always want to help and please.*
They **SEEK** to have their **CONFIDENCE** boosted from friends.

AFFECTIONATE – like to have their tummy tickled

Strong affinity for   **throat**
                                  female reproductive system
                                  ovaries
                                  breasts

Good for RHEUMATISM, SCIATICA

Very good remedy for **tonsillitis**

** SYMPTOMS GO FROM RIGHT TO LEFT, AND BACK AGAIN **
(e.g. in a sore throat)
LIKE A DOG WAGGING ITS TAIL

HEADACHES from right to left and back again

Better for a WARM DRINK
Better for drinks in general

Feels worse for swallowing nothing, empty swallowing

Swollen glands

Lac Caninum

FOOD:

Loves MILK
Loves **PEPPER**
Loves *SPICY FOOD*

Dislikes SWEET THINGS
Aversion to LIQUIDS, especially WATER

Voracious appetite all the time (*"canine hunger"*)

Good MENSTRUAL remedy:
Women who get a sore throat with their period

Sore breasts, especially pre-menstrually
- < JARRING
- < **TOUCH**
- < **cold air**
- < *wind*
- < *draughts*

Erosion of the cervix *(also Creosotum)*
Ovulatory pain

Heavy periods – red, profuse and hot

Helps dry up breast milk in women who want to stop breastfeeding
Also balances the flow.
   [General rule: use Lac Defloratum to PROMOTE breast milk, & Lac Caninum to DRY UP]

Lac Caninum

Lac-C is most similar to Lachesis, Arg Nit and Pulsatilla

Sore throats
Ovarian pain
Sore breasts
Snakes
BUT mentally very different

Sweet-natured
Desire to please
Affectionate
Likes open air
Menstrual problems

History of promiscuity
High sex drive (libido) – *"like a dog on heat"* (*cf. Pulsatilla, Lachesis* - often use their sexuality to get love and affection)
Desire to please boyfriend

[Most 'land animal' remedies have a high libido]

Barking coughs!

                        Worse after sleep (also Lachesis)

Placid, but can flip over into ANGER, AGGRESSION

Lac Caninum

- snappy - but will regret it later.

Doesn't harbour a grudge

Vertigo
FEELING OF FLOATING IN AIR (Can have 'out of body' experiences)
Clairvoyance possible

Very sensitive people
  Fear of thunderstorms (not strongly so)

Orderly people – *not allowed to express themselves*

Main points:
Lack of self-confidence
Sense of self-doubt
Fear of, or dreams of, snakes
Dislikes draughts (also Lac Defloratum)
Right-Left alternating – *like a tail wagging; also the changeability of a Pulsatilla*

Lac Defloratum

Skimmed (cow's) milk

Not as big a remedy emotionally as **Lac Caninum**
For NUTRITION and BLOOD; Heart; Head

Used mainly:
- To stimulate breast milk
- Lactose intolerance

Mentals:

Horror of having doors closed
Claustrophobia – won't go in a lift

Feels forsaken
Lots of sadness
Suicidal depression

Easy exhaustion, whether or not active

Lack of NUTRITION
Children thin, undernourished
Don't assimilate well
Tired and anaemic

ICY FINGERTIPS

Feels like cold air blowing on them
Feels like sheets are damp
Ill effects of loss of sleep
Dizziness, especially on turning in bed

Lac Defloratum

Vertigo on closing eyes

STRONG AVERSION to MILK
Good for babies who reject milk
Aggravated by milk if they drink it.

VOMITING IN PREGNANCY

Persistent CONSTIPATION

Chilly, cold, especially fingertips

Very sensitive to *cold*

Can't bear the light
PHOTOPHOBIA
Headaches from light

Related remedy: Natrum Muriaticum

	Summary:
1	**Milk (agg. and aversion to)**
2	Claustrophobia
3	Malnourishment
4	**Complications of pregnancy**
5	*Chilly – icy extremities*

Lilium Tigrum

Tiger Lily

HYSTERIA, over-reaction

Not <u>yielding</u>, but not <u>aggressive</u>
'Hot, sexy Sepias'
Highly sexed
So **HOT** they can look flushed, cyanotic

Delusions that people have done something wrong to them:
takes things the wrong way (*cf. Platina – haughty, refined, idealistic person who's become disillusioned and now feels superior*)

Prolapses, especially uterine
Pushes down onto vagina and makes them easily excitable

Retroverted uterus

Feels aroused most of the time – *because of the pathology*
Feels nervous about this because of ethical beliefs: ∴
    tries to DISTRACT HERSELF

Becomes HURRIED; strong sense of <u>URGENCY</u>

Must keep BUSY (*cf. Sepia – 'occupation ameliorates'*) – to
    be diverted and repress sexual desire
Everything is **rushed**

Miscarriages

Lilium Tigrum

Have HIGH STANDARDS
Have a conscience
Create lots of work
WILL SIT AND FIDGET
'Full of tormented rush'
Snappy, *irritable,* worse from consolation

Occupation ameliorates

Tries to CONTROL – everything is in a whirl

Theatrical nature ⎱ Unlike Natrum
Loves to be the centre of attention ⎰ Muriaticum

Passionate about whatever they're doing – especially
   religion
Feel guilty and **remorseful – TORMENTING THOUGHTS**

WILD, CRAZY feelings in the head (*cf.* *Medorrhinum*)
Gets *irritable* (→ liver)

CONSTANT DESIRE to go to the lavatory

Burning palms and soles *(concomitant)*

Staphysagria is also quite highly sexed – but Staph's suppress their emotions and express themselves through sex. **Lil-T is highly sexed because of bearing down on the uterus –** <u>*pathology*</u>

Lilium Tigrum

Food: aversion to COFFEE, BREAD
       desires MEAT

[Fraxinus Americanus tincture is a drainage remedy – tones up the uterus]

Warm, and busy - *cf. Apis*
Desire for PHYSICAL EXERTION, which ameliorates

Worse 5 – 8 p.m.

Male genitalia – complaints from suppressing sexual desire

> PRIESTS

Tension between sexuality and morality.

Alternating symptoms: womb/heart/mental symptoms

Cf. Platina – the sexiest remedy in the Materia Medica

Right sided (unusually) heart symptoms

Luna

ARRESTED PUBERTY

Issues, problems left over from puberty - never been well since puberty.

First love

Menses very irregular, only a few times a year.

Lack of female development, small breasts etc.

Reproductive incapacity

The pineal gland is responsible for the major cycles. This gland is very sensitive to light and dark. If luna *fails, try* pineal gland *as a sarcode (a remedy made from healthy tissue)*

> You can give the affected part in potency - it draws the body's healing powers to the part like a homing device. The body doesn't know where the problem is.
> The more pathological the case is, the more difficult, the more benefit you'll see from the use of sarcodes.

VIVID DREAMS
Wakes unrefreshed

Stuck – unmotivated to do anything
People get stuck when they're shocked - dissociated from the pain.

Angry – irritable, towards own children
Totally fed up with her life (*cf. Sepia*)

Luna

OUTBURSTS of anger, with tears

Confused
Dazed
Can't concentrate
"FLOATY"

THIRSTY, unusually so – particularly for cold drinks

Can't tolerate alcohol
Gets terrible **hangovers**

Pre-menstrual Syndrome – PMS

Dysmenorrhoea

Headaches: changeable, *cf. Pulsatilla*
Headaches worse at menses

Dry **EYES**
    DRY skin
        Dry **NOSE**
            Dry LIPS
                Dry **THROAT**

Eyes get SORE, itchy, **tired**

Lyssin

Also called *Hydrophobinum*.
Made from the saliva of a rabid dog.

A very SYPHILITIC remedy

FEAR OF WATER
Other hydrophobic remedies: Stramonium, all of the Solanaceas - Belladonna, Hyoscyamus; Cantharis

MANIC
HYPERSENSITIVE TO EVERYTHING AROUND HIM
RAGING

A strong sense of having been **tormented** all the time - *SEETHING* because of the constant torment.

Practically **beside themselves with rage**
(*cf. Staphysagria. Lyssin doesn't have a nice, sweet side.*)

Sense of dependency – *cf. Stramonium* - can't leave the relationship (doesn't have the courage to go) and **explodes** occasionally into **violence**
Followed by **remorse, sorrow,** *regrets*

Like the dog - *has an owner*, is *dependent* on the owner, even if the owner is cruel to them. Just **SNAPS** every so often - FEAR is there. Fear of going away, of diving into the unknown.

one of the first remedies for
** AGORAPHOBIA **

Also **Claustrophobia**

Lyssin

The most **extreme** state of the animal nature - fear of water - fear of over 80% of the substance of our own composition.
Fear of **HEARING** water, running, trickling
Can't **drink** water

Locked into an emotional world that's tormenting them - feelings are **HEIGHTENED, <u>HYPERSENSITIVE</u>**
Heightened **senses** - **sound**, SMELL, sense of **pain**, light

At **breaking point** - can't bear any more.
<u>Not</u> sensitive to the feelings of others - it's a personal, selfish hypersensitivity.

A major **ABUSE** remedy - for someone who's now **raging against the world**
Can **become** the abuser, the tormentor - **MANIPULATIVE**, *HYPER-NERVOUS*, **VERY ANGRY**

Sense of **ABANDONMENT**, being **FORSAKEN** (*cf Pulsatilla, Stramonium*) - utterly alone, abandoned in grief and sadness. Sense of **betrayal**, **FORSAKENNESS**, isolation (like the treatment of a rabid dog)

Sensitivity even to a breath of air on the skin.
Fear of **BRIGHT OBJECTS** - light glistening on the water (*cf Stramonium*) - sends them into a rage.
Can be thrown into **convulsions** even thinking about water, light, the heat of the sun

Lyssin

Other fluids don't have the same effect as water.

Craves chocolate

RABIES
Never been well since **RABIES VACCINE**

Consider also for **bites** - of dogs, snakes

A feeling that the wound has healed <u>too quickly</u> - poison was locked in too soon. *The rabies wound heals very quickly.*

PARANOID FEELING OF BEING WRONGED

Delusion of having been **abused, betrayed**
(cf Hyoscyamus)
Reaction is **violence**

(Keynote) Every so often they will flare up into an **EXPLOSION OF RAGE**, followed by **REPENTANCE**. *(cf Anacardium - but Anacardium doesn't "feel")*

Can turn to **drink**

They look **WILD**, slightly **CRAZY**

Hate the rain *(cf Naja, Elaps)*
DON'T LIKE BATHING

Intense, *charismatic*, MANIC

Lyssin

Very **SEXUAL** remedy - sometimes completely out of hand especially in the male

Inability to ejaculate

Sometimes he will have night ejaculations, but is unable to climax in sex.
A *MANIC* quality to their sexuality

Ailments from sexual suppression (for males) – (*cf Conium*)

Brahmacharia, in India:
Like a coiled spring

Constantly **MOVING**, *RESTLESS*, **WILD**
Seething energy

Compare: Lac Caninum has a sense of self disgust, having been put down, beaten. Another dog remedy.

Longing for a state of safety

RAGE, **anger**, *violence* inside the person is generally directed at the person they're dependent on.
A very disturbed Staphysagria.

Sensitive to **heat**, COLD, bright lights, *water, draughts of air*
The sensory barometer is at its peak
Delusion of being a dog
Can **growl** when they express themselves - a constriction in the throat *(cf. Drosera)*

Lyssin

Wants to **mutilate** himself *(cf Mercury, Syphilinum)*
Wants to **SLASH HIS WRISTS**, stub cigarettes out on his arm *(cf Hyoscyamus, Arsenicum)*

Has a dreadful self image

Sense that something **AWFUL** is going to happen to them. *The pain they are going to inflict on themselves is better than the pain they are going through by living*

They can become very **critical, ABUSIVE**, tormenting themselves.

Can **commit suicide**
Can also beg people to **kill** them - to end it all
Have *two trains of thought occurring at the same time*, in conflict with one another *(cf Anacardium, Naja)*

SCHIZOPHRENIA

Intense, alive, *quick thinking* (when not in manic phase)
Can easily **tip over the edge**
They think they're going **MAD**

Can turn to religion, fanaticism - endlessly praying, beseeching *(cf. Veratrum Album)*

RITUALISTIC, **COMPULSIVE** behaviour (to give a sense of safety) *(cf Arsenicum, Iodum)*

Lyssin

Obsessive behaviour

Episodic - can be affected by the moon

"Anxiety when hearing church bells" (*religious guilt*)

Sighing
SPASMS in the throat
Constant **SALIVATION** - thick, stringy *(cf Syphilinum, Mercury)*
Difficult to speak: can't express themselves -
   as if they're choking *(cf Ignatia)*
Stuttering, choking, SPASMODIC *(cf Mercury)*

Physical symptoms:
   Abscesses
   Boils
   Pussy **eruptions**
   Feeling that they want to tear, stab the eruptions.
   Tearing at the self because of the torment of skin eruptions
   "*If I let it out, it will be better*" - a need for, but an **inability to express**
   WOUNDS HEAL quickly, becoming **BLUE, SORE, INFLAMED**

   Glandular **swellings in axilla**, and in **groin**
   Bloody, mucousy **stools** with **spasms**
   Constant DESIRE TO URINATE - particularly when hearing RUNNING WATER
   Great sensitivity of the genitalia (men and women)

Lyssin

BREASTS very **SWOLLEN**, tender, **SENSITIVE** to touch

Can **prolapse** *(cf Sepia)* - everything collapses into insensitivity

One of the *first remedies* for '**Never been well since**' ... **a bite, poisoning, wound** etc. where *Ledum* would be given as the acute remedy

A feeling in the head as if it's **light** and **floating**
Hair becomes **thick, MATTED, OILY**
Excruciating **HEADACHES** - often at the back of the head, as a result of a bite
Cf. Belladonna - headaches, sensitive to light, water fear, mania

Craves **SALT**
Craves **chocolate**
Prefers **warm drinks** to cold

DELUSIONS:
 of **ANIMALS**
SEES *dogs*
 sees animals
THINKS HE'S A DOG
 of *being insulted*
 of *being injured*
DREAMS OF FIRE - THEY'RE BURNING INSIDE
DELUSION that they're something special - great person - a **PARANOID** side

Magnesia Carbonica

MgCO$_3$ Magensium Carbonate
"The Orphan's Remedy"

A **TUBERCULAR** remedy
An under-proven remedy
Loss of ability to assimilate food and nourishment
Emaciation

Soured
JAUNDICED } attitude to life
Oversensitive

Bowels, and stomach

Stool like whitish clay, or spluttery and green (*cf. Colocyncthis, Chamomilla*)

Nervous
Restless
Irritable

Pale
Drawn
Feels abandoned, forsaken
Dreams that he's lost in his own house

Children who get behind at school, are unable to develop writing skills

Magnesia Carbonica

Withdrawn from life
Sad and taciturn

> Sensitive to the least touch – *starts when touched*

Unable to assimilate LOVE

They lack the material base – the paternal element – of the Carbon

Dependent on CARE, **SECURITY** and *SUPPORT* (and feel they have none)

Suppressed emotions
ANXIOUS, desperate, all the time,
No secure roots
Must move about

Unrefreshed after sleep
> walking in open air

FOOD: CRAVES MEAT, fruits, acids, vegetables
     < MILK
     Sourness: smell like sour milk

Heavy, bloated abdomen

Magnesia Carbonica

COLD, CHILLY
 Children don't thrive – they stay THIN,
  weak, *UNDERNOURISHED*
Irritable children

Menstrual symptoms:
 Menses mainly flow **at night**
  - only flow when there's no pain
  - only flow during sleep.
 Sore throat before menses

Eyes: **Black spots, cataracts**

Sudden **DEAFNESS**

 Someone who says "*I never dream*"

Sharp, shooting pains along the nerves, esp. of FACE and TEETH
Toothache, < at night
  cold air
  change of weather
  pregnancy

Magnesium Muriaticum

MgCl₂ Magnesium Chloride

The keynote picture, according to Scholten:
Magnesium is a FLARE, a flash of light, fireworks.

Quick burst of energy, then it dies down quickly.

∴ all Mags have CRAMPS, SPASMS

All Mags also have intense PAIN (so e.g. Magnesium Phosphoricum – period cramps)

The 'Muriaticum' element introduces the 'mother' aspect.
'Muriaticum' also indicates
        FEAR of LOSS
        PAIN of LOSS (e.g. pain of parents fighting)
        AGGRESSION – OR NOT (do I fight, or become a pacifist?)

MAG Mur pathologies lie in the NERVOUS SYSTEM and LIVER
because of constant fighting around them, and they desperately want to bring the warring persons together.

Mag Mur – 'The Peacemaker'

Magnesium Muriaticum

More *genuine* than Lycopodium
[Mag Carb = "The Orphan"]

Not cowardly, or selfish in motives

Child (8 – 10 years) develops **liver pathology** because he's surrounded by aggression.
As the child grows, he develops a ***jaundiced,*** sour attitude to life.

Dislikes confrontation – realises the futility of fighting

Feels **despondent, pessimistic.**

Can WITHDRAW FROM LIFE (*cf. Natrum Muriaticum*):
"You go to the party – I'll just be a drag if I come along"
(and they're probably right!)

Delusion that they don't have any friends (also Sarsparilla)
BUT PEOPLE LIKE AND RESPECT THEM

Have taken on too much, and have been hurt:
→ *sour attitude*, withdrawal

Magnesium Muriaticum

Feeling that people they put their trust in will betray that trust

Can't allow themselves to have a friend – they'll be let down

Hysterical women – losing their grip emotionally

Liver pathologies: chronic enlargement, jaundice
Low energy

Allergic reactions
** inability to digest MILK **
** can't digest SALT ** *gives them gastritis*
(Also Natrum Muriaticum)

** Aggravations from the SEA **

Tremendous LONELINESS
Abandoned, forsaken

Irregular **BOWELS** (constipation or diarrhoea)

Very catarrhal
  mucus, phlegm
    especially
    - anywhere near *salt*, or *the sea*
    - *in bed* at night
        (feels obstructed, can't breathe)

Magnesium Muriaticum

Wake in the morning feeling worse than when they went to bed.
They gradually feel better during the day

All Mags **DREAM OF FIRE**
(think of the magnesium flare)

Burning, spasmodic pains
Neuralgic pains
Period cramps
endometriosis
protracted, painful periods
ACNE & SPOTS around menses

Almost MANIC DEPRESSIVE

Dreams of ROBBERS
Dreams of the DEAD
Dreams that she's lost

Kleptomaniacs – and they steal *dainties* (they want a treat)

Very sensitive – has taste (*as with Natrum Muriaticum*)
Self-awareness, arising out of suffering

Self-consciousness

Manganum

Mn — Manganese

Affinity for: **ear, nose, throat** and **larynx**

Action on nervous system produces improvements lying down as generality. So specific ailments are also improved by lying down.
Feels better lying down.

Tiredness
CATCHES COLD EASILY
Often anaemic
Worse for humidity, cold,(before storms), cold air
Better for **SMOKING CIGARETTES** (e.g. because it's cold)

Clears throat all the time
Cough with hoarseness, usually from humid cold

Overuse of voice → cough

> ★★PATIENT GETS A SPASMODIC COUGH IF HE SCRATCHES THE INSIDE OF HIS EAR★★

Laryngitis: pains radiating to the ears
Chronic running nose

Smallest cold goes to the chest
Oblomov's syndrome:
Goes to bed – the only place they

Manganum

feel well

Metal manganese is the metal of RESPONSIBILITY
(Magnesium = flightiness)

Manganum patients will need manganese-rich food.

Certain drugs (e.g. hallucinogens) demolish manganum.

FULL OF IDEAS

Not making the transition to the real world.
Not necessarily spacey.
A foggy mind, but won't be aware of it

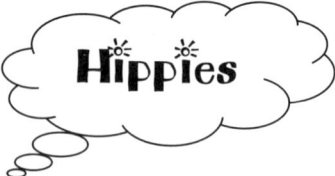

Hippies

**Hippy who lies around in bed all day smoking.
60's flower power**

HEY MAN - YEAH, FAR OUT!

Non-responsible behaviour has become embedded into the values of contemporary culture: legislation is needed where once there were personal / social restraints.

> Parents who leave children at home while going on holiday
> Forgetting to pick child up from school.

Manganum

Usually men, sometimes women

A single dose of manganum 200c may suffice. If patient is still on drugs, manganum can be antidoted. This is highly individual, however, and manganum can still be prescribed even through drug-taking.

Manganum may be found in an unmaternal mother *(Aetiology of sensitivity to anaesthetics, gas, during birth process?)*
Can be used post-natally (especially if drugs, anaesthetics, were used)

In **anaemia**, if ferrum is indicated and hasn't worked, try manganum as well

'Soft' drugs: don't interfere with social function immediately. *However they still change the body's chemistry, demolish memory and attention span.* Acute and chronic poisoning occurs

ECSTASY, LSD poison the system quickly; cannabis less so.

Hallucinogens suppress suppressions, make you 'feel good'.
Prozac does the same.
AMPHETAMINES AFFECT FITNESS OF THOUGHT.

Manganum

Drugs can make bodies stupid

Prolonged cannabis use induces long-term poisoning: users get high on the excitement of ideas, which don't turn into reality.
Sulphur is close to manganum in this, but

> Sulphur avoids the issue
> **Manganum avoids the responsibility of that issue**

Morgan is the relevant bowel nosode (where there is a strongly indicated nutritional component - the bowel is often at the root of the problem.)

Morgan
Morgan Pure (Paterson)

Keynote: CONGESTION

Associated with the **PSORIC** MIASM.
Used where the patient is **SLUGGISH** and
CONGESTIVE.

Affects the **PORTAL SYSTEM**: diseases of the
liver, gallbladder

bronchitis
congestion
weight gain
** *menopause* **

cholesterol blockages

OBESITY

associated remedies: **SULPHUR**, SEPIA,
GRAPHITES, PETROLEUM,
CALC CARB,
LYCOPODIUM

SKIN PROBLEMS: ECZEMA, ITCHING, REDNESS, PSORIASIS

(Try Padma 28 – a herbal antioxidant - for arterial blockages)

Headaches before periods

Morgan
Morgan Pure (Paterson)

Congestive headaches

CALC CARB – for hypothyroidism – putting on weight; also gallbladder.

> *It is said.... Give Calc Carb 10m on a full moon for weight loss*
> Give Silica on a new moon

Florid complexions: redness of cheeks, lips.

TENSE, NERVOUS STATES;
depressed, irritable, weepy

Bronchitis, especially in winter

Dry, burning throat –parched.

Cracks in the corners of the mouth

Swollen tongue, raw, red
Dry, cracked lips

Catarrh

Otorrhœa

CONJUNCTIVITIS
Styes

Morgan
Morgan Pure (Paterson)

Iritis

Acne rosacea

Fibrositis

Lumbago
Pains are better for HEAT, *moving*, or at start of movement
Rheumatism - in hands, sacro-iliac, shoulders.
Joints are swollen and painful

HUNGER PANGS AT 11A.M.

Heartburn
Vomiting, nausea

LIVER and GALLBLADDER:
Jaundice
Gallstones
Headaches relieved by VOMITING

Circulatory problems:
varicose veins
PHLEBITIS
VARICOSE ULCERS

Morgan
Morgan Pure (Paterson)

CONSTIPATION
Pruritus
Itching of anus or genitals

Cystitis

Insomnia
Restless sleep

Sweaty armpits

Eruptions on the face, behind the ears
Cracks, fissures
Weeping, itchy, scaly

Acne

Burning

ITCH, ITCH, itch

Flat warts on the hands
Chilblains
Erythema

Varicose eczema

Morgan Gaertner
(Paterson)

A variant of the Bacillus Morgan bowel nosode.

Related to **Lycopodium**

Aggravates at 4 – 8 p.m.

Anxiety, irritability, apprehension

'LIVERISH' tendency

Affinity for **urinary tract**:

> Renal colic
> **Renal stones**
> Kidney infections
> CYSTITIS
> *Vaginitis*

FLATULENCE
PSORIASIS

Respiratory problems

Impatient
Tense

RESTLESS
Depressed
Jealous
Fear of crowds

Morgan Gaertner
(Paterson)

CLAUSTROPHOBIA
Nervous breakdown

Nail-biters

Alopecia

Facial neuralgia

Blepharitis
    Styes
        Cysts on eyelids
              CORNEAL ULCERS

Nasal catarrh
Sinus problems

Polyps in nose

Otitis

Bitter taste in mouth

Pyorrhoea
Recurrent TONSILLITIS

ASTHMA
Ticklish cough

Tightness of chest

Morgan Gaertner
(Paterson)

Intercostal neuralgia (pains between the ribs)
Desires: **SWEETS**
      Salt
      Fat
      Eggs
      Meat
      Hot food

Averse to: **FAT**
      Eggs
      Meat

Distended feelings
Indigestion, with belching
Constipation
Piles
Anal fissures
Pruritus

Gallbladder pains
Cholecystitis

Arthritis, in shoulder, knees, wrists, elbows

Sweaty feet

Naja

The Cobra   Naja Tribudians

Symbol of serpent **power**, *kundalini*, the awakened earth

A **noble** creature ("King Cobra")
Qualities of *nobility, responsibility, morality*

Najas feel that in some way they've suffered wrong, leading to **brooding** (*cf. Hyos)*, **melancholy wallowing** (*cf. Pulsatilla)*

Rubric: **Broods over imaginary troubles**

Physical problems arising from a snakebite:
Lachesis: wound becomes septic
Naja: you hardly notice the bite, but victim almost <u>drowns</u> in his own body fluids – **wallowing, mentally and physically**

Oedema

Water elements - ∴ *cf. Pulsatilla*

Morbid, brooding, suicidal tendency (*cf. Aurum*)

Irresolution - alternating moods

SPLIT – feel they have two wills
      Schizoid tendency – (*cf. Anacardium*)

Feels neglected, uncared for

Naja

Retains the SNAKE quality that they're **UNDER SUPERHUMAN CONTROL:**
They can believe that they're in contact with something higher than them.
Pathologically, can HEAR VOICES

They have an identity crisis: "Who am I?"
Oedema, water, brooding → ****FEAR OF RAIN**
** *(also Elaps)*

** **heart problems** **

especially
 ** **heart valve problems** ** *(#1 remedy)*
 (also Strophanthus)

Nobility – reverence and fear (a split) (as with snakes)

Can have a FEAR OF SNAKES

The caduceus – symbol of mercury, the British Medical Association, Society of Homeopaths: Also represents the sympathetic/parasympathetic nervous system

Constriction and dryness of the throat – Suffocative feeling in the larynx

There is a PLAYFUL side to this remedy:

Naja

- *frivolous*
- *playful*
- *happy*
- *jolly*

        (but not often)

Najas are not light, trivial people

(cf. Lilium Tigrum) a connection between HEART, OVARIES, and UTERUS

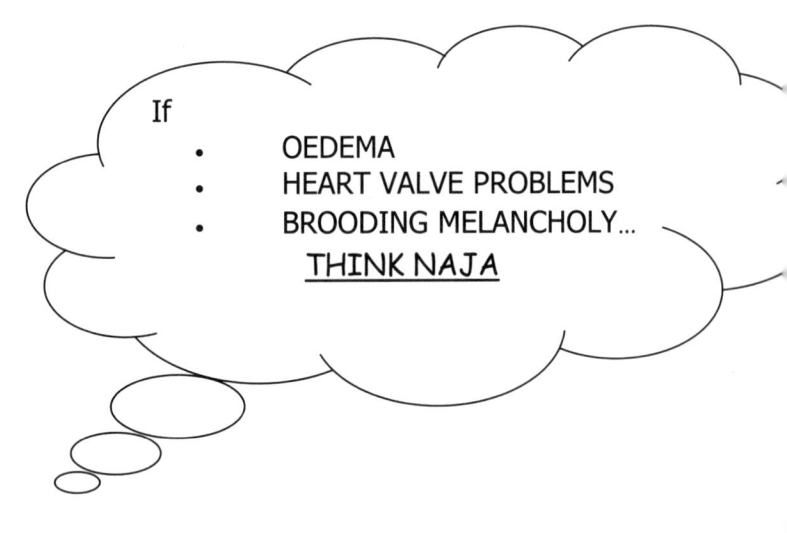

If
- OEDEMA
- HEART VALVE PROBLEMS
- BROODING MELANCHOLY...

    <u>THINK NAJA</u>

Clairvoyant tendency

Naja

MODALITIES:

< ** lying on left side **	> WALKING
cold air	*riding in open air*
rain	lying on right side
ALCOHOL	
pressure of clothes	
after sleep	
AFTER MENSES	
touch	

Most BACK PAINS are upper back / thoracic

Bladder: uneasiness / pressure in bladder
Red sediment in urine

Tendency to
    Mottling of skin (*because of circulatory problems*)
       - *not as extreme as Lachesis*
    Purple/livid colour

Itching scars

Natrum Sulphuricum

Nat Sulph

Glauber's Salt (a purgative)

No delusions are listed in repertories for this remedy.

Why?

Either

NO IMAGINATION,
or
an inability to give yourself a 'get-out' - a dream, fantasy, escape from the ugly reality of life
Nat Sulph is **GROUND DOWN BY THE PRESSURES OF LIFE**.

Suicidally depressive - *cf. Aurum* - **by shooting, or hanging**

*They **will** actually kill themselves (they don't have a let-out)*

Mental troubles from a head injury - especially to the back of the head (occiput)

A **SYCOTIC** remedy

CHEERFUL AFTER STOOL *(cf. Borax, other Natrums)*
Will evacuate a huge amount.

Weighed down with water - **a 'sponge' remedy**.

Very **earthy**

Natrum Sulphuricum

*Star sign is **Taurus***

MENINGITIS

WORSE IN WET, HUMID WEATHER (<cold or hot damp)

Ascites *(puffed up abdomen full of water)*
Bowel accumulates a tremendous amount of water
- a fluid imbalance
Flatulent, windy

A **LIVER** remedy
Gallbladder problems
BILIOUSNESS
NAUSEA

Urethritis
Suppressed **gonorrhea**

A major **PHOTOPHOBIC** remedy

BITTER taste in the mouth
Foods: desires cold drinks, **salty fish, beer**
desires, or averse to, **YOGHURT**
Averse: **meat**, bread

ASTHMA, < early morning, especially ca. 4 a.m.
 humid asthma
 Give with Thuja when Arsenicum fails in Asthma

Whatever they do, nothing succeeds

Natrum Sulphuricum

systematic workers, down to earth
not **spontaneous**
objective and **realistic**

Gurgling, rumbling in gut

Spluttering, wind, in stool
YELLOW, LOOSE STOOLS
Sulphur goes to the loo before breakfast; Nat Sulph goes to the loo after breakfast.

For gallstones, or as a liver flush:
fast for approximately 6 hours from midday; take 1 tbs Epsom salts in ½ pint water; repeat in 2 hrs; 2 hrs later drink 100mg of olive oil with a squeeze of grapefruit juice; go to bed; in morning, take another tbs epsom salts and repeat 2 hrs later.

This will act as a great purgative and will help eliminate gallstones

China, cholest, carduus marianus, chelidonium, nat sulph, in low potency, will help soften gallstones.

Nitricum Acidum

Nit-Ac   Nitric Acid

HATRED to a person who's offended them and unmoved by apologies

Very **UNFORGIVING**

Delusions they're engaged in a **law suit**
DAGGERS DRAWN, ALL THE TIME

Suspicion, **HATRED**, **barriers put up**, and constantly in **DISPUTE**

Embittered, hateful feelings

(Think of TNT – explosives – contain a tremendous force of [destructive] energy)

**ANXIETY ABOUT THEIR HEALTH **
   predominantly CANCER

Suspicious nature refuses to accept others' advice

RESENTMENT AGAINST THE WORLD

In the early stages, they are also SYMPATHETIC

An amazing friend, and an appalling enemy

Starts off lively, bubbly, effervescent and then moves towards **COLLAPSE**

Nitricum Acidum

AILMENTS FROM NIGHTWATCHING.

Exhaustion

Always feel **threatened**;
- in health
- in work
- IN RELATIONSHIPS

Never feel secure, happy

*When Nit-ac walks into a room it becomes a battleground. They bring **arguments in their wake**.*

Never satisfied with what you say.
Won't believe you.

They feel that survival depends on them being **HARD**, **cold**, **distant**, **scornful**, cruel (*cf. Scorpion*)

Feel **CUT OFF, THREATENED**

Physically:
Affects areas where the mucous membranes and skin join:
- Mouth
- Eyes
- Anal fissures
- Splits / tears in genitalia
- Genitalia – often bleeding, painful

Nitricum Acidum

If they pass a stool there is agony for hours afterwards (*they have, and are, a pain in the bum!*)

Acrid, staining vaginal discharge

Splitting
Cracking } **ACIDIC QUALITIES**
Burning

<u>WARTY</u> – painful and bleeding (soft, spongy warts are Thuja)

Dreadful <u>ACNE</u> – on back and face;
Painful – almost malignant

Hypochondriacs, in a positive state early on, but later become **negative**

Aggravated by consolation, being spoken to

Very **COLD** people

Obstinate

Raging energy

Cf. Mercury and Thuja: both **syphilitic** and **sycotic**

Splinter-like pains

Nitricum Acidum

One of the first remedies for
BOWEL CANCER
(*also RUTA*)

Incredibly impetuous

VIOLENT, ANGRY, MALICIOUS – *trembling* with anger

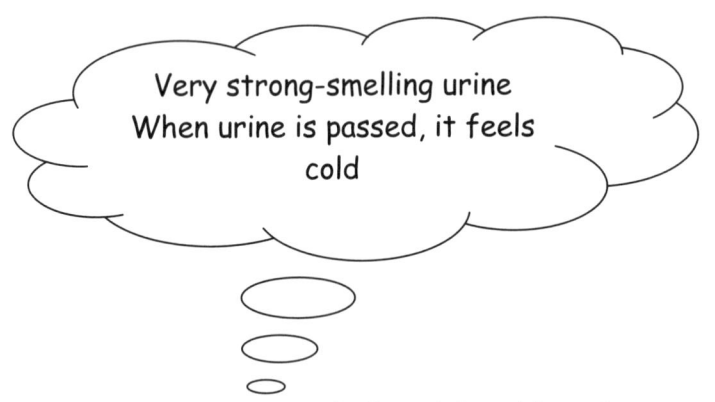

> Very strong-smelling urine
> When urine is passed, it feels cold

Many symptoms around genitalia and the genito-urinary system: pains, burning, discharges, acridity, spots, lumps, chancres, ulcers, etc. etc.

LEUCORRHŒA

A **CHILLY** remedy

Compare ANACARDIUM – hatred, cursing, violence

Nitricum Acidum

Food Symptoms:
  Butter

  Pork scratchings!

  Craves BUTTER
  Craves FAT (*cf. Hepar Sulph*)

  Aggravated by milk
  They like **lemonade** (real)

Opium

A Narcotic drug
                Morphine and Heroin are derivatives

Narcosis, sleep, dream-inducing (Cocaine: 'awake'-inducing)

Good especially for **children** and **the elderly**

Desire to escape from body.
Endorphins – pain dampeners – are released in the brain.
We are drawn to the opiates because we want to escape the pain of modern life.

Key symptoms: **PAINLESSNESS**
(*cf. Helleborus*) where we'd expect pain.

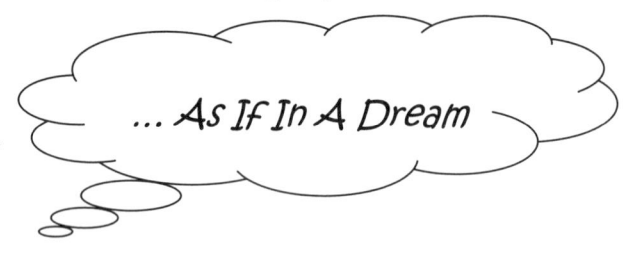

> ... *As If In A Dream*

Consciousness-changing
A DREAMWORLD

Scared of reality, the 'here and now'

> *Romantic poets*: Coleridge, '**Kublai Kahn**'

Opium used to be sold as **LAUDANUM**.

Opium

Used in aetiologies of **TRAUMA**, shock, FRIGHT, **car accident** – jerked out of the self and stuck there.

As if life has passed them by – no life experience shows on the face

Never quite recovered from anaesthetic

Nothing quite functions – bodily functions have shut down, asleep

Sleepwalking – *SOMNAMBULISM*

SNORING
                Altered perceptions

Alcoholics
People who've been on drugs

They never show fear

Makes fantastic life plans, but doesn't live it out – the dream remains a fantasy

#1 remedy where **bowels are seized up** (after drugs, surgery, in the elderly)
    no pain, but nothing moves. *No peristalsis.*

INTUSSUSCEPTION in babies (*also Plumbum*)

Drifts into a *comatose state*
    on a life support machine (*cf.* Carbo Veg, Camphor)

Opium

YAWNING

Also the opposite:
- *epilepsy*
- **pain**
- TREMBLING
- JERKINESS
- convulsiveness
- rage
- desire to kill

ABORTION AS A RESULT OF FRIGHT

Never been well since (NBWS) fright

retention of urine after confinement

HOT, all over
ITCHING

<	emotions fear FRIGHT **odours** **ALCOHOL** suppressed discharges WARMTH sunstroke	>	**COLD** uncovering (head)

Opium

Aetiologies:
fear
FRIGHT
ANGER
shame
alcohol
lead poisoning
sun

Petroleum

ROCK OIL
A LONG CHAIN OF HYDROCARBONS

A major **SKIN** remedy

Very similar to Graphites
made out of **PETROL**.
Dirty, **HARD**, **ROUGH**, parchment-like skin
Skin is **RAW**, FESTERS, won't heal

Worse in the **folds of the skin**
Eczema

DEEP CRACKS

Eruptions which are thick and hard.

Aggravated by **cold**
Itching and **burning**
   Patient scratches until he bleeds

Mentally, a very **excitable**, **quarrelsome**, **irritable** patient
one of the most **irritable** people around.

Worse from alcohol

Irresolution
   Indecisiveness

Petroleum

Loses his way in well-known streets (*cf Aluminum, Mercury*)
Confusion walking in open air

Sense of DUALITY
thinks he's someone else, or a limb is double.
Feels close to death

emotionally, close to the **LIVER**, and
GALLBLADDER (paired channels in acupuncture)
Anger (Liver)
GALLBLADDER has the emotion of *indecisiveness*.
Many remedies featuring *indecisiveness* have
GALLBLADDER problems (*Calc carb, Graphites, Pulsatilla*)

Petroleum has as a concomitant to skin GASTRIC PROBLEMS.

MOTION SICKNESS
CAR SICKNESS
Nausea with gastric problems

OFFENSIVE PERSPIRATION
INCREASED mucus - lots of CATARRH
Psoric and sycotic miasms

BLEPHARITIS

Petroleum

> "The Greek Lorry Driver"
> (Vithoulkas)
> *putting petroleum jelly on their hands all the time*

Dryness of skin
Generally CHILLY

Feet perspire; *smell is so strong you can smell in the next room* (cf Graphites)

Injuries slow to heal (cf Graphites)

Phosphoricum Acidum

Phos-Ac   Phosphoric Acid

Phos-Ac's love **refreshing** things – **lemonade**

A sympathetic, empathetic, <u>caring</u> person who's been worn down by caring for others.

Ailments from GRIEF

Picric Acid	-	Intellectual Exhaustion
Phosphoric Acid	-	Emotional Exhaustion
Muriatic Acid	-	Physical Exhaustion

<u>Utterly wiped out</u> emotional state of someone who's cared for a person dying of a terminal illness

Totally drained – can hardly speak
(*Natrum Mur* – *closed, holding in;*
Ignatia – *hysterical;*
Phos Ac – *totally wiped out* – *no emotions left* – *the plug has been pulled*)

Slow; refuses to answer questions – can't answer: there's nothing there anymore.

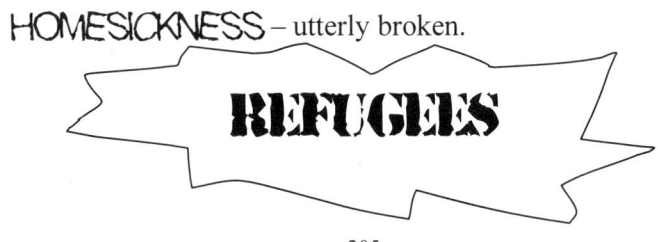

HOMESICKNESS – utterly broken.

REFUGEES

Phosphoricum Acidum

Struggle, followed by collapse.

Loss of hair, or going **grey** overnight, from
GRIEF

AILMENTS FROM CARE

Can't summon up any (emotional) energy – they brood, become interned.

A short sleep revitalises them
TEENAGERS – first love – feeling lost
Exhausted, apathetic state
Pining away
Totally inert, thin, **anorexic**
Refuses to eat:
Anorexia

Diabetes – with an emotional connection

Totally **dehydrated** – sometimes also **thirstless** as well as thirsty

Craves **refreshing things** e.g. **fruits**

Painless, watery diarrhœa that increases dehydration but doesn't appear to create debility

ailments from humiliation, *mortification*, being **put down**

Platina

Pt   Platinum metallicum

In the *periodic table*:
the **pinnacle** in the 6th line (the '**leadership line**') of the periodic table.

Most **egocentric** remedy of the entire *materia medica*.
Most **precious** of all metals.

Most **PROUD**
Most **HAUGHTY, ALOOF**
Most **CONTEMPTUOUS** OF OTHERS

"IT'S LONELY AT THE TOP" – Platina's dilemma

cf. Pulsatilla: delusions they're alone in the world
           isolation
           feeling of abandonment
           but because they're so
           <u>*special*</u>*, the 'best'*

Delusions they're bigger than they really are
Will misjudge **distance** – e.g., distance of stairs

Walk, gait is very upright, regal, dignified

OUTRAGEOUSLY SEXUAL

Split in make-up:
     THINKS HE'S THE BEST
     ON TOP OF A MOUNTAIN

Platina

also **INCREDIBLE (ROMANTIC) IDEALS**

hypersexual – base chakra

Difficult to reconcile the two.

ARROGANT, DISMISSIVE

Sexual energy can be deviated and channelled into

HAUGHTINESS INFLATED EGO

or vice versa

Doesn't want to compromise

CULT LEADERS
(with Pulsatilla, Lac Caninum *disciples)*

DYNASTY:
Alexis Colby
(Joan Collins)

Platina

A very SYPHILITIC remedy – as are all the 6th line remedies in the periodic table (5th line is more SYCOTIC)

DESTRUCTIVE – *sees a knife and has an urge to use it*

Everyone is beneath them (*cf. Veratrum Album: "it's a god-given thing"*)

**Hears voices
under superhuman control**

Cold, alone, desperately isolated

Aversion to children – *because children don't recognise their airs and graces:*

The Emperor's New Clothes

Sense of BEING BORN INTO THE WRONG FAMILY
hasn't ended up where he should have been

Many **sexual complaints** especially **female:**
uterine, ovarian problems
sexually hypersensitive
or
numbness of the part

Platina

> **SUMMARY:**
> Egocentricity
> **CONTEMPT FOR OTHER PEOPLE**
> **split** between **ideas & sexuality**
> **HYPERSEXUALITY**

*Platina is used in catalytic converters in cars: is this a contributing factor in the rise of road rage? ("get out of my way – don't you cut me up" – **arrogant, egocentric** rage)*

> in open air – *not restricted*

Masturbation at a very early age: early sexual awakening

An only child who's much adored: *products of the Chinese policy on one-child families?*

Nothing lives up to their romantic ideal

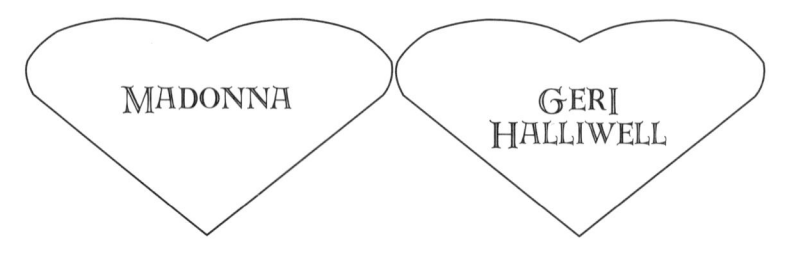

MADONNA   GERI HALLIWELL

Lilium Tigrum (religious affections alternating with sexual excitement)– antidoted by Platina- blown up out of all proportion

Proteus

The **BRAINSTORM** bowel nosode

Used when there are prolonged periods of stress and strain.

Imbalances in the central and peripheral nervous systems

Symptoms appear SUDDENLY

An EXPLOSIVE remedy

OEDEMA
Spasms
Cramps
Menstrual Problems
EPILEPSY
Duodenal ulcers

The "FRIGHT – FIGHT – FLIGHT" response: the autonomic nervous system

Perspiration, pumping heart, edginess – ready to go

Sudden increase or decrease in the blood supply

For disturbances of the chloride metabolism.
An affinity for the KIDNEYS
The kidneys are sited next to the adrenal glands. Chlorine is produced, leading to an imbalance. Chlorides → MURIATICUM remedies.

Apprehension
FEAR

Proteus

Anger
The system suddenly goes out of kilter

> **Related remedy:**
> **NATRUM MURIATICUM**

Loners
Not violent
Keep their grief to themselves

They can **EXPLODE**, even commit murder
Tantrums

> **3 acutes of Natrum Mur:**
> **Ignatia** *(not thirsty)*
> **BRYONIA** *(extreme thirst, can't move)*
> APIS *(busy all the time)*

Muriaticum issues: mother, nurturing, home
    Kali Mur: issues of responsibility, duty etc. around nurturing, home life
    Calc Mur
    Aurum Mur
    Ammonium Mur
    Magnesium Mur: spasms; angry, fiery about mother. Very depressive. Children of parents who quarrel. Aversion to violence. Make peace among others. "The Peacemaker"

Proteus

Magnesium types have a great affinity to Proteus – fiery, impulsive, explosive
Muriaticum types are **PEAR-SHAPED**

Related remedies: STAPHYSAGRIA, COLOCYNTHIS, CAUSTICUM
(Staph internalizes anger (goes to liver, gallbladder); Causticum becomes a revolutionary)

Proteus is THIN
Emaciated

Sudden, frontal HEADACHES
HEADACHES before periods
MIGRAINES
Burning pains
Acute pains

(Give PHOSPHORUS for anyone who doesn't come out of anaesthetic well)

ANGINA – *due to spasms of coronary capillaries*
DUODENAL ULCERS – *where there are no preceding symptoms*

For **ANGIONEUROTIC OEDEMA**: *APIS (acute of Natrum Muriaticum and a kidney remedy)*

HERPETIC ERUPTIONS
Sudden cold sores around the lips, mouth, eyes

Proteus

Someone who talks very fast

Carcinosin in low potency, also Kali Phosphricum, can calm down the nervous system (a good sleeping remedy)

Drainage remedies associated with Proteus:
*Avena Sativa ϕ, **Passiflora** ϕ.*
Passiflora ϕ is also particularly useful in cases of epilepsy.

Fibrous **thickening**

Dark haired types; thin; pale

Chronic arthritis

Meningitis

RAYNAUD'S SYNDROME

Menière's disease (vertigo)

Fluent coryza

Mouth ulcers
SALTY TASTE IN MOUTH
CRACKS in corners of the mouth

Fibrositis, especially in the neck, head.

Phlebitis

Proteus

> *Averse* to pork, **butter**, boiled eggs, **green beans**, onions
> *Desires* eggs, **fats**, sweets, salt
> *Gets* upset by **eggs**

FLATULENCE, ABDOMINAL PAINS

Dupuytren's contracture

Intermittent claudication

Muscle cramps (*cf. Cuprum Metallicum*)

Diarrhœa alternating with constipation
Stools yellow, soft

    Piles, itching and bleeding

        Dermatitis
        Pruritus
Sweaty armpits: **BOILS** in the armpits

Worse: on waking, in the morning
      from **exertion**
      from **HEAT**
      from **EXPOSURE** – to the sun, or to cold in the winter

Aggravated by WINE

Ranunculus Bulbosa

Buttercup

A **shingles** remedy
Shingles with **burning pains** which remain after they have gone.

Stitching, tearing, agonising pains (*as in pleurisy*)

STORMY, rainy, **wet weather** aggravates them appallingly. (*cf Rhus Tox*)
Worse for weather changes

A chilly remedy

HEADACHES, rheumatic problems, NEURALGIC PAINS (*also Rhus Tox*)
    Differentiation: Rhus tox is **better for** movement; Ranunculus bulbosa is **worse for** movement)

INTERCOSTAL PAINS (between the ribs), *especially neuralgic*

Alcoholic tendency - **CRAVES ALCOHOL**

ALCOHOLICS

CONFUSED mental state

IRRITABLE
'LEAVE ME ALONE - I DON'T WANT TO MOVE'

ANGRY

Ranunculus Bulbosa

Quarrelsome (alternating with a caring tendency - *cf. Pulsatilla*)
Abusive

Concentration difficult - vacant feeling

Cowardice
A coward who turns to drink to give himself 'Dutch courage'

FEAR of work
FEAR of being alone (*cf Staphysagria*)
FEAR of **change**
FEAR of GHOSTS (*cf Staphysagria*)

Wallowing in self pity

THINKING OF THEIR COMPLAINTS AGGRAVATES

people who **talk to themselves**

Faintness before eating - needs to eat.

Storminess, CHANGEABILITY, yet they need to be still, stable. **Aggravated by change.**

Better for eating **PORK** and **BACON** (*also Tuberculinum, Rad Brom*)

Saccharum Officinalis

Sugar Cane

SUGAR is an addictive drug.
It has no food value – it causes *de-nutrition* – leaches nutrients out of the body.
Closely related to **Carcinosin**

History:
It was peddled throughout the British Empire: along with tobacco, opium, tea, coffee. Imperial conquerors provided these drugs as crops for their vanquished territories. Deception is a part of the essence of this drug.

Today, 25% of all calories consumed come from SUGAR. These are often hidden in processed foods.

DECEPTION
Unlike Mercury or Thuja, this is SELF-deception: the patient cuts himself off from the truth about HIMSELF – how he feels, who he is.
DENIAL

Sugar is used as a PACIFIER, and to TRICK people: it makes BITTER things ACCEPTABLE.

Sugar pacifies BABIES and YOUNG CHILDREN: it goes deep into their psychological and physioloigcal beings

Sugar is a **SUBSTITUTE** for **ATTENTION**, comfort, **LOVE**
It NUMBS FEELINGS

Saccharum Officinalis

Sugar is a method of **REWARD** and **PUNISHMENT**

Self-judgement

Terrified of anger – can't cope
People who build a WALL against all emotions (*cf. Natrum Mur*), especially ANGER
Emotions (joy, anger) rise and fall- like peaks and troughs of energy. Without this movement of feeling, when emotions are blocked, it can create a physical pathology.

A *MASK* – "everything's okay".

AILMENTS FROM SUPPRESSED ANGER (GRIEF, DISAPPOINTMENT)

SECRETIVE
LIARS
People who never show how they feel (but will tell you their physical ailments)

An extremely high pain threshold

Dissatisfied
Quarrelsome
Whining and complaining
Irritable
Oversensitive
Fidgety
OUTBURSTS OF VIOLENT TEMPER
Indifference

Saccharum Officinalis

A SYPHILITIC remedy

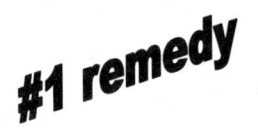

#1 remedy for BREAKING ADDICTIONS (*heroin, tobacco, alcohol, junk food…*)

Hyperactive children

Depressed immune system
Mental depression (*from suppressed emotions*)

Acidity – decayed teeth
Mouth ulcers
BLEEDING GUMS
Cracks in tongue

Glaucoma
Cataracts
DIMNESS OF SIGHT

M.E.
CANCER
Thrush, candida
PMS *(pre-menstrual syndrome – irritability, depression before menses)*
Weak, pale menses – suppressed flow or incredibly heavy
Suppressed discharges

Gallstones

Saccharum Officinalis

Irritable bowel syndrome

Malnutrition
ACNE – Ulcers – slowness of healing

HYPERGLYCAEMIA, HYPOGLYCAEMIA
Diabetes
Pancreatitis

Calcium deficiency (*sugar leaches minerals from the body*)

Osteoporosis
Glands, liver, spleen,
arms/legs/face swollen

ANOREXIA

BULIMIA

BLOATING
SWELLING
OEDEMA

Acid stomachs
Constricting feeling in the abdomen

Vomiting white, sour mucus; hungry

High blood pressure
Cardiovascular disease

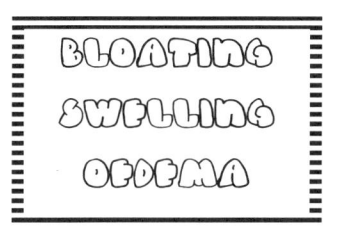

Sanguinaria

Blood Root

A member of the papaver group - also Chelidonium, Opium.

The **pain relief** *of sanguinaria is similar to the pain relief of the opiates.*
Right sided **CERVICAL PROBLEMS**, going up and over right side of head to right eye and right shoulder

Chelidonium has an affinity with the **gallbladder**; so does Sanguinaria, even though its major **pathology** is in the **blood**.

Acrid, dark red discharges
SCALDS and **BURNS**

Hay fever symptoms:
Dry nose, with congestion
Right-sided *nasal polyps*
coryzas
headaches
RHINITIS
Burning in the larynx, nose, throat
CHEST HOARSE, WHEEZY, ASTHMATIC
Palms and soles of feet dry, red-hot, wrinkly

bursitis
Liver problems

GALLBLADDER problems

Sanguinaria

ROSE COLD (sensitive to the smell of flowers) (especially in June) - **main remedy**

Wakes up with a headache which gets worse during the day.
NAUSEA and VOMITING
Migraine
VOMITING WITH HEADACHES, feels better for vomiting
DIGESTIVE DISTURBANCES

Mucous membranes: **DEEP, CHESTY SYMPTOMS**
Will **COUGH** constantly, ending with a loud **BELCH**

Sticks feet out of bed *(cf. Sulphur)*

A cold remedy

Craves spicy food (*cf Sulphur*)
FEELS BETTER FOR EATING SPICES
Ameliorated by sour things

Spigelia

Pinkroot
Wormgrass

A member of the *loganacea* group:
NUX VOMICA, IGNATIA, GELSEMIUM, SPIGELIA, CURARE

Named after a botanist - Dr. Spigelius

Affects the *nerves*, HEART, **EYES**, teeth, **fibrous tissue**

> ** **GREAT FEAR OF NEEDLES, PINS, POINTED OBJECTS**
> (*cf. Silica*)**

HORROR of **inoculations**

PAINS - agonising, nerve-like

Left-sided headaches - "like a nail"
Agonising headaches that **go into the eyes**

> **Aversion to tobacco smoke**

Sighing
SENSITIVITY (*cf. Ignatia*)

For SERIOUS, SENSITIVE PEOPLE with SERIOUS PAIN. (Vithoulkas)

The focus for Spigelia is in the **cervical nerves of the neck**. Can lead to **nerve damage**.

Spigelia

TRIGEMINAL NEURALGIA in the face

Left sided bursitis
Left sided shoulder pains

Heart pathology - *pains going down the left arm to the little finger*

Refined, delicate people
Right brained - *intuitive, artistic*

Low **pain threshold**
They feel pain very **intensely** - pains are **VIOLENT**
COLDNESS of the painful parts

Stammering
chilly
sensitive to TOUCH

(**A WORM remedy**)

(think of PIN WORMS) *also Cina, Absinthum, Artemis vulgaris*

BOWEL PROBLEMS

Facial **nerves**, cardiac **nerves**, are affected

Spigelia

Irritation, anger (*cf. Nux Vom*)

Eye symptoms: a major eye remedy.
Eyes are constantly changing their focus:
   prescription changes frequently

Worse in the daytime

Heart and eye symptoms combined
Neuralgia
Glaucoma of the left eye

Stitching pains around the **heart**
like a needle has been dug into the nerve tract

Angina pectoris

A FIRE remedy

Much worse for tobacco (*cf Ignatia*)
Aversion to COFFEE (*cf Nux Vomica*)

Sulphuricum Acidum

H₂SO₄   Sulphuric acid
Sul-ac

HURRIED, RUSHED combined with EXHAUSTION

Lots of energy, apparently – can't stop

BUT the tank is empty – no reserves of energy.

URBAN DWELLERS
    Hyperactive, but with no real energy
    Stuck in a traffic jam: getting nowhere fast

> Burnt out, but can't stop

Weak
Exhausted

> **ill effects of urban pollution**

Nervy, hyperactive, agitated, exhausted *as a result of urban pollution*

Will look **cool, detached, urbane** – has an inability to connect on a deep level.
Superficial relationships
A **surface remedy** – not deep

ULCERATION
    Mouth ulcers

Sulphuricum Acidum

Drugs and drink *(cf. Quercus)*
Dislikes water unless it contains alcohol

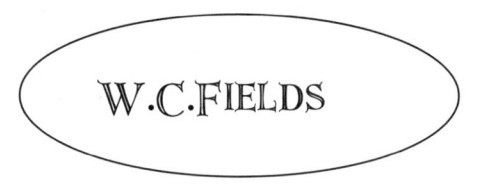

(W.C.FIELDS)

Chilly: hot flushes bring out a cold sweat

Face will go <u>red</u> during a hot flush

Compelled to go faster *(cf. Mercury [look for ulcers and <u>trembling hands</u>])*

> SEASHORE
< **Smoke, fog, pollution**
    hates industrial areas

SCARS have a tendency to redness

Sour perspiration
    Sour belching
        Sour **breath**
            A <u>sourpuss</u>
                Sour taste on vomiting
    HEARTBURN

Stools are <u>yellow</u>

Sycotic Co

A bowel nosode

Related to Medorrhinum, Thuja, Tuberculinum

Keynote: **IRRITABILITY**

Affects the *mucous membranes, lymph glands*

Catarrhal conditions
Discharges are **yellow-green, thick**

PALE, ANAEMIC TYPES

Puffy faced, especially under eyes and in the morning
Fat, flabby

Nervous, **tense, ANGRY** people

Restless, weepy, *depressed*, shy, **exhausted**

NAIL-BITERS
Warts
Oily skinned people

FEARFUL of **animals**, dogs, **the dark**, being alone

Similar in mental state to GAERTNER
Sycotic Co. children try to hide their fear more than Gaertner children.
Gaertner types are thin, undernourished; Sycotic Co.'s are **fat, flabby**.

Sycotic Co

Fearful and irritated – outbursts of temper (*cf. Lycopodium*)

Measles-like or **varicella-like** rash

Conjunctivitis
 Photophobia
  HEMIOPIA

DEAFNESS
Otorrhœa

MENINGITIS
CONVULSIONS
Epileptic seizures

Irritation of the meninges

Chronic, deep-seated headaches.
Headaches from a sinus infection

Throbbing headaches, lasting for days or even weeks.
Left-sided headaches.

Often headaches are **worse during menses.**
Head sweats at night.

FURRY TONGUE
Deep *fissures* on the tongue
Overgrown tonsils and adenoids
Recurrent *tonsillitis*

Sycotic Co

RAW, DRY, SORE FEELING IN THROAT

Profuse **mucus in throat** in the Morning (*cf. Kali bichromicum*)

Asthma and **bronchitis**, better at the sea-side, worse for damp

> Wheezing, COUGHING.
> Spasmodic coughing 2 – 3 a.m.
> Croupy cough at night.
> Can cough until they VOMIT

Influenza, catarrh – give Sycotic Co. to *prevent recurrence*

Generally worse 2-3 a.m.

Pleurisy

Fibrositis

LUMBO-SACRAL PAIN

Pain BETTER FOR MOVING, BETTER FOR HEAT

Fussy in eating habits

Averse to:
egg, **FAT**, dairy products, SALT, sugar, **vegetables**, tea

Upset by: **onions**, ORANGES, **FAT**

Sycotic Co

Can't eat breakfast
Nauseous at the thought of eggs (*cf. Ferrum*)

IBS – IRRITABLE BOWEL SYNDROME
Leucorrhœa

Warts, condylomata around **anus**

Used in canine distemper, cat flu, foot and mouth disease, foul pest, as well as human influenza.

Tarentula Hispania

Spanish Wolf Spider

"LIKE A COILED SPRING"
INDUSTRIOUS
Workaholic – 18 hours per day
Full of energy – like they're on a drug

(FOREIGN EXCHANGE (FOREX) WORKERS)

Phenomenal **reserves of energy**

SPINAL PROBLEMS
Manic dancing – dancing the imbalance out of the system

(Air Traffic Controllers)

Rhythm ameliorates
horse riding
music
massage
DANCING

233

Tarentula Hispania

Frantic, CRAZY, HYSTERICAL

In the gym every day

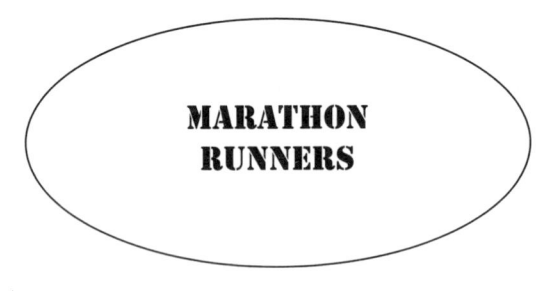

> MARATHON RUNNERS

Probably an imbalance in the lower centre – a **blockage**
Very **material**

ANIMAL CUNNING - gut feelings
(no higher insight)

Cunning

Hysterical while being watched
HYPERACTIVE, MANIPULATIVE, CUNNING CHILDREN

Aetiology: ill effects of unrequited love

LOVE MUSIC, COLOURS (*attracting a mate*)
Love to make a show – make themselves **noticed**

> **Music** (*also aurum*)
  Tarentula: **ROCK MUSIC**,
  Aurum: *classical music*

Tarentula Hispania

Better for being industrious (*also aurum*)

FEAR OF BEING TRAPPED, HIT, ASSAULTED – leads to avoidance

Desire for **OPEN AIR**
Sexual erethism (fast) - very sexual
Very sensitive genitals

Sensitive to the *least touch*: averse to being touched
< *Touch*, > **rubbing**

CAN'T BEAR TO BE TOUCHED ON THE SPINE

Foxy, SLY, **magnetic qualities**

Suddenly violent, DESTRUCTIVE, *impulse to do harm*

Jerking motions
TWITCHING
JUMPY

Tarentula Hispania

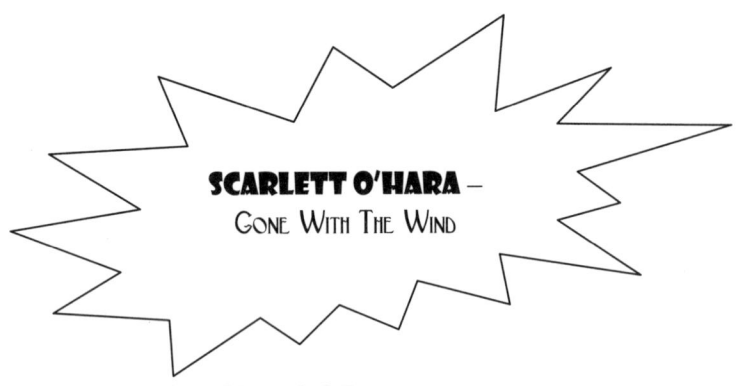

SCARLETT O'HARA –
GONE WITH THE WIND

Craves SPICY FOOD
Averse to **MEAT**, bread, chocolate
Desires **COLD DRINKS**, salt, raw food

refuses to eat

Rolls from side to side to relieve

Chilly, but **DESIRE FOR OPEN AIR**

Veratrum Album

White hellebore

'Being right' is at the centre of this remedy.
It's the *pathology* of being right.
Kent thought that Veratrum Album would remove half the lunatics in the asylum.

A remedy used in the **cholera** epidemic during the Napoleonic wars.

Veratrum has the **cholera** picture –
   severe digestive disorders.

Extreme symptoms - not for little things.
For example: *unbelievable agony* with periods!
Similar to arsenicum album – has the same intensity – you can DIE from your symptoms.

PAINFUL DIARRHOEA:
   In children
   girls at puberty,
   really painful periods with diarrhoea, vomiting,
becoming cold, **BLUE LIPS**, cold sweat, **COLD with cold sweat**. (*cf.* Arsenicum album: *burning pains*)

Headaches,
   great **violence**,
      coldness,
         VOMITING OF BILE,
         exhaustion,

Veratrum Album

retching on an empty stomach.

ICY COLDNESS of the entire body.

LIKE COLD WATER RUNNING THROUGH VEINS

Beads of cold sweat, especially on forehead.

SEVERE food poisoning: complete collapse with extreme coldness.
(*Also Carbo Vegetabilis, Arsenicum*)

Everything is VIOLENT AND SUDDEN

Sensation as if **ICE** on vertex.
SENSATION OF COLD WATER TRICKLING

May be **incoherent** or even **unconscious**

Desperately thirsty for **ICED water**, for **ice cubes**. *Makes them colder, but doesn't stop the craving.*

Wants to be covered. *Lack of vital heat means covers have no effect.*
Frequent **GUSHING DIARRHOEA** with **EXCRUTIATING ABDOMINAL PAINS**
Dehydration from diarrhoea

Completely constipated
No peristalsis

Veratrum Album

Stools: **hard, round, black balls**. (*cf. Opium*)

Period pains
Endometriosis, with NAUSEA, vomiting, **FAINTING**

Extreme reaction to *pain*

MIGRAINES

Sciatica

RAYNAUD'S SYNDROME

Insanity
Temporary insanity brought about by
SUPPRESSION, fevers, **eruptions**, POISONING,
injury with **extreme shock**

Aetiologies of FRIGHT, disappointed love, **mortification**, *wounded honour*

LOQUACIOUS,
GESTICULATING
crazy

The Joker
IN
BATMAN

Excessive smiling, foolish mirth, hilarity.

RIDICULOUS GESTURES

Kisses everyone in sight

Veratrum Album

DELUSIONS:
OF HAVING CANCER
OF BEING IN LABOUR
THAT THEY WILL LOSE THEIR PLACE IN
SOCIETY - *causes despair*
  That they are a **great person**
  (Napoleon, Jesus Christ)

ACUTE, COMPLETE INSANITY
WILD
  VIOLENT
    DESTRUCTIVE
    Biting
      Kicking
    THRASHING
    Tearing clothes off in fury
  Desires to escape and run away

Loquacity is – lewd, sexual (good comedians)
  LASCIVIOUS
  sexual mania

Indisposition to talk
Despairing
Refusal to touch anyone
Feeling FORSAKEN
Suicidal
  WANTS TO JUMP FROM A WINDOW, OR
    DROWN HIMSELF

Often highly critical and censorious of others.

Veratrum Album

People who preach in the streets:

REPENT! THE END OF THE WORLD IS NIGH!

Sense of righteousness

THINKS HE'S THE ONLY ONE WHO IS SANE, AND EVERYONE ELSE IS MAD

High mental energy, yet physically depleted
(cf. Stramonium - insanity comes with vastly increased physical strength)

Veratrum Album is the

pathology of certainty

Zincum

Zn   Zinc

Very like Phosphorus

Affinity for BRAIN and NERVES
BLOOD

FRIENDLY, OPEN PERSONALITY

MENTAL PROSTRATION - total cerebral exhaustion. Brain fag (*cf. Pic-ac*)

Inability to **THROW THINGS OFF**

There is a profound deficiency in zinc - because of the incidence of NERVOUS RESTLESSNESS, SPEED, EXHAUSTING, HYPERACTIVITY. Also from depletion of the soil and of the food we eat.

STRESS   **Can't sleep**
Can **SLEEPWALK**, sleep**TALK**, **TOSS AROUND IN BED**
Can't relax in spite of tiredness
Will **shout out** in sleep
PARANOID DREAMS (of being pursued, 'got at')

Emotionally cold
cut off from feelings (*unlike Phosphorus*)

Hypersexual, but *cerebrally so*

GUILT –
    I've done something wrong –
    I M GOING TO BE ARRESTED

Zincum

CHANGEABLE, ALTERNATING MOODS
Irritability
NOTHING SEEMS RIGHT

Yielding

Constant complaining – *whinge, whinge, whinge*

Menopause
Reproduction and fertility -
   PROSTATIC DISORDERS (*also Selenium*)
   ejaculate has a high level of zinc
sexually out of balance - giving sex too much importance, or
                  no importance
               sexually exhausted
(*cf. Pic Ac, Kali Phosphoricum*)

Trembling
Convulsive state, TWITCHING from
the suppression of a discharge - skin eruptions
Suppression of **ECZEMA**, SWEAT - goes directly to the
nervous system

*Children are often naturally **intellectual**, **striving**, and are pushed to the point of **exhaustion**.*
Feeling of HAVING TO PERFORM - **pressured** by
parents in order to perform intellectually

Zinc is a **NERVE NUTRIENT** in the same way that
Ferrum is a **BLOOD NUTRIENT**.

An ingredient in nappy rash creams, in plasters.

Zincum

One of the first remedies for nappy rash (and **anal itching** in adults… as a result of **suppression** of **nappy rash**?)

Zinc sits next to Copper in the periodic table (column 12). Cuprum and Zinc are both **convulsive** remedies - a stop-start **convulsive tendency**.
- Cuprum is more DRAMATIC, EXPLOSIVE, or completely suppressed;
- Zinc is a constantly AGITATED, nervy state.

Failure to achieve → **GUILT**
sense of persecution
NERVOUS WRECKS before examinations
NOTHING IS ABLE TO BE THROWN OFF. Inability to discharge

Never been well since a skin eruption

N⁰ ENERGY
OVERSENSITIVE TO NOISE

No discharges, fevers when ill

May have headaches, **bladder** problems
ENURESIS

In extremis leads to **EPILEPSY**
CUPRUM FOR GRAND MAL; ZINCUM FOR PETIT MAL

Zincum

HEADACHES:
sensation of pressure
> hard pressure;
< warmth

> Horrible things, sad stories, affect them profoundly

GREAT AMELIORATION DURING MENSES
Better for secretions, flow of menses (cf. Lachesis, but Lachesis has more energy)

Restlessness, especially of **legs**

Calcium, magnesium zinc, for men with **prostate problems**

COOL, detached, **intellectual**
no emotional reaction
A BLANK FACADE
Talks about **DEATH** dispassionately, without fear or feelings

In later life, Parkinson's disease (the mask)
Motor Neurone Disease
(*also* **Curare** - *main vegetable kingdom remedy, with* Gelsemium, *for Parkinson's, Motor Neurone disease*)

TORMENTS EVERYONE WITH THEIR COMPLAINTS:
(*because nothing ever clears up they've always got something wrong with them*)

Zincum

Can occasionally have an **EXPLOSION** - of **rage, upset**

> **Keynote: even a sip of wine gets them very drunk,** accompanied with nausea, headaches, red face, bowel upsets**

Very sensitive to **pressure** on the nervous system
> eating - *shakes with weakness from hunger*
⊂⊃ **WINE**
< sweets - *cause heartburn*

Gets **ravenously hungry** around 11 a.m. or 12 p.m.
**exhausted, sinking feeling around 11 a.m.

Averse to **FISH, meat, sweets**

Index

A

AAA, 23
Abandoned, 38, 131, 162, 168
Abandoned
 fear of being, 72, 207
Abdomen
 bloated, 104, 118, 169
 distended, 33, 60
 pains in, 86
 pot belly, 109
 something alive in, sensation of, 50
 swollen, 57
Abortion, 200
Abrupt, 142
Abscesses, 112, 120, 166
Absent-minded, 52
Absinthum, 225
Abuse, 131, 162
 history of, 103
Abusive, 87, 121, 142, 165, 217
Acids
 craves, 169
 desires, 123
Acne, 132, 174, 195, 221
Acne rosacea, 181
Aconite, 64, 119
Acrid, 12
Active, 99
Addictions, 220
Adenoids
 overgrown, 230
Adrenal glands, 211
Affectionate, 150
Agaricus, 44
Aggressive, 99, 171
Agitated, 227, 244
Agnus Castus, 48
Agoraphobia, 149, 161
Air, 14, 103
 open air, 18
Air traffic controllers, 233
Alcohol, 67, 75, 200, 202
 alcoholics, 132, 199, 216
 craves, 216
 intolerance of, 160
Allergies, 107, 109, 173
Alone
 fear of being, 46, 98, 217, 229
 wants to be, 82
Aloof, 207
Alopecia, 100, 184
Alternating symptoms, 28
Aluminum, 203
Alzheimer's Disease, 116
Ambra Grisea, 68
Ammonium, 12, 117
Ammonium Carbonicum, 11
Ammonium Muriaticum, 17, 212

Index

Amnesia, 115
Amoral, 53, 83, 99, 132
Amphetamines, 177
Anacardium, 21, 83, 163, 165, 186, 196
Anaemia, 59, 92, 143, 154, 175, 229
Anaesthetic, 117
  effects of, 199, 213
Anarchists, 13
Ancistrodon mokeson, 52
Angel on one shoulder, devil on the other, 24
Anger, 13, 55, 98, 159, 161, 212, 216, 229
  excessive, 121
  terrified of, 219
  violent, 142
Angina, 106, 213, 226
Anhalonium, 26
Animals
  fear of, 229
Anorexia, 59, 145, 206, 221
Anthrax, 39, 47
Antibiotics
  never been well since, 111
Anus
  anal fissures, 185
  itching, 244
Anxious, 31, 45, 51, 85, 89, 102, 131, 169, 183
  health, about, 193
Apathy, 26, 72

Aphasia, 39
Aphrodite, 77
Aphthae, 29, 145
Apis, 77, 158, 212
Appetite
  easily satisfied, 14
  increased, 51
  voracious, 151
Apples
  aversion to, 118
Apple-shaped, 18
Apprehension, 211
Argentum Nitricum, 90, 148, 152
Armpits
  boils in, 215
Arnica, 116, 124
Arrhythmia, 86, 94
Arrogant, 135, 208
Arsenicum Album, 15, 36, 53, 90, 110, 113, 125, 165
Artemis vulgaris, 225
Arthritis, 70, 81, 95, 185, 214
Artistic, 58, 80, 110
Ascites, 191
Assaulted
  fear of being, 235
Asthma, 88, 93, 123, 132, 143, 146, 184, 191, 222, 231
Aurum, 11, 85, 97, 138, 186, 190, 234

Index

Aurum Muriaticum, 212
Authority, 12
Autism, 115
Autumn, 88
Avaricious, 70
Avena Sativa, 108, 214
Axilla, 215
   glands swollen, 120
   sweaty, 182
   swellings in, 166

B

Back, 62
   pain, 19, 93, 109
Bacon
   better for, 217
Bag ladies, 70
Ball
   sitting on a, sensation of, 50
Band
   around the parts, 24
Baryta Carbonica, 47
Bathing
   dislikes, 163
Bed
   fear of going to, 49
Bed-wetting, 244
Behaviour
   compulsive, neurotic, 126
Belching, 185
   need to, 30
Belladonna, 60, 77, 87, 161, 167

Benzoic acid, 28
Berberis Vulgaris, 30
Betrayed
   sense of being, 162
Bigger
   delusions he is, than he really is, 207
Bile, 59, 76, 129
   vomits, 237
Birth
   difficult, 35
Bite, inclination to, 45
Bites, 112, 163
Bitter, 12, 23, 59
Black, 74, 97
   wears, 81
Bladder, 48, 189
Bleeding, 95
Blepharitis, 34, 92, 122, 184, 203
Blindness, 39
Blood, 11, 14, 17, 74, 112, 124, 128, 146, 222, 242
   difficulty with coagulation, 39
   in mouth, taste of, 30
   poisoning, 112
   pressure, 85, 221
   throbbing, 53
   transfusion, 58
   vessels, boiling sensation in, 20
   vomits black, 39

Index

Blue babies, 35
Boils, 112, 120, 143, 166, 215
Bonding
 difficulty with, 106
Bones
 degeneration of, 100
 pain at night, 143
Borax, 31, 145, 190
Bothrops, 38, 118
Bowel nosodes, 35, 211
Bowels, 168, 173, 199, 225
Brahmacharia, 164
Brain, 242
 brainstorm, 211
 damage, 45
Brain fag, 79, 91
Brave, 172
Bread, 109
Breastfeeding
 stopping, 151
Breasts
 cancer, 46
 lumps, 142
 pains, 35, 104
 sensitive, 167
 shrivelled, 126
 sore, pre-menstrual, 151
 swollen, 167
Breath
 foul, 145
Breathing, 13
 irregular, 86
 shallow, 27

 worse lying down, 35
Bright objects
 fear of, 162
Brilliant objects
 aversion to, 47
Bromine, 125
Bronchitis, 122, 179, 180, 231
Brooding, 186
Bruises, 14, 95
Bryonia, 36, 212
Bubbly, 99
Buboes, 47
Bufo, 44
Bulimia, 221
Bullying, 55
Burning, 15
Burn-out, 79, 227
Burping, 94
Bursitis, 222, 225
Butter, 109
 craves, 195
Buttercup, 216

C

Caduceus, 187
Calcarea Carbonica, 31, 33, 47, 77, 87, 98, 111, 179, 203
Calcarea Muriatica, 212
Calcium deficiency, 221
Calendula, 113
Camphor, 117, 199

Index

Cancer, 66, 110, 220
  bowel, 196
  breast, 46
  delusions of having, 240
  fear of, 148
Candida, 104, 220
Cannabis Indica, 26, 48, 178
Cantharis, 161
Car sickness, 69, 111
Carbo Vegetabilis, 117, 199
Carbonicum, 12
Carbuncles, 47
Carcinosin, 102, 103, 214, 218
Care
  lacks, 169
Cashew nut, 21
Castaneda, Carlos, 26
Cataracts, 71, 170, 220
Catarrh, 32, 88, 119, 122, 144, 173, 180, 184, 203, 229
  crusty, 97
Catatonic, 114
Cats
  dislikes, 149
Caustic, 12
Causticum, 13, 117, 213
Celandine, 55
Celibacy, 67, 78
Cenchris Contortrix, 52
Censorious, 87, 240
Certainty

  sense of, 241
Cervix
  dilation of, 63
  erosion of, 151
Chamomilla, 36, 110, 168
Change
  aggravated by, 217
  fear of, 217
Charismatic, 53, 163
Cheese, 108
Chelidonium, 55, 222
Chemotherapy, 110, 117
Chest, 13
  infections, 88
  tight, 184
Chilblains, 109, 182
Childbirth, 63
  delivery slow, 65
  post-natal, 177
Children, 35
  aversion to, 209
  beat, desire to, 55
  dirty, 14
  disobedient, 14
  fostering, 149
  indifferent to his, 140
  love of, 149
Chilly, 14, 18, 53, 121, 225, 228
China, 57, 83
Chinchona, 57
Chlorine, 125
Chocolate, 14

Index

craves, 163, 167
Choking
  as if, 166
Cholecystitis, 185
Cholera, 237
Cholesterol, 179
Christmas Rose, 114
Church bells
  anxious when hearing, 166
Cigarettes
  better for, 175
Cimicifuga, 62
Cina, 110, 225
Circulation, 11, 14, 181
  ailments of, 95
Cirrhosis, 75
Clairvoyant, 38, 50, 72, 153, 188
Claudication
  intermittent, 215
Claustrophobia, 154, 161, 184
Clergyman's throat, 123
Clothing
  tight, aggravates, 73, 75
  tight, aversion to, 53
Cobra, 186
Cobwebs
  sensation of, on face, 32
Cocaine, 198
Cocculus, 69
Coeliac disease, 109
Coffea, 36
Coffee, 29, 71

aversion to, 226
Cold, 24, 237
  ailments from exposure to, 88
  catches easily, 175
Cold sores, 213
Cold weather
  better for, 33
  damp, worse for, 33
Colds, 88, 92
Colic, 14, 33, 60, 79, 89, 128, 146
  renal, 183
Colitis, 94
Colocynthis, 79, 168, 213
Colour
  noise, touch seen as, 26
Colours
  loves bright, 38
Coma, 199
Company
  aversion to, 98
Complains constantly, 243
Complexion
  florid, 180
Compulsive, 165
Concentration
  difficult, 89, 160, 217
  poor, 116
Conception, 35
Condylomata, 123
Confidence
  lack of, 21
Conformist, 108

Index

Confrontation
    dislikes, 172
Confused, 89, 103, 160, 216
Congestion, 179
Conium, 66, 84, 164
Conjunctivitis, 92, 180, 230
Consolation
    worse from, 157
Constipation, 81, 124, 137, 155, 173, 182, 185, 199, 238
Constriction, 30, 38, 46
Contemptuous, 207
Contracted, 77
Contradiction
    intolerant of, 121
Control, 24
    fear of losing, 49
    feels controlled by another, 105
    feels under superhuman, 187, 209
Controlling, 87
Convulsions, 80, 131, 146, 162, 230
Cooking
    loves, 80
Copperhead Snake, 52
Coral Snake, 97
Corneal ulcers, 184
Coryza, 214, 222
Cough, 88
    barking, 123, 152
    constant, with belching, 223
    hoarseness, with, 175
    scratching ear causes, 175
    spasmodic, 175, 231
    ticklish, 184
    wheezing, 231
Covered
    wants to be, 238
Covetous, 70
Cowardice, 217
Cracks
    deep, in skin, 202
Cramps, 211
Cravings
    food, 103, 108
Crazy, 234, 239
Creative, 80
Creosotum, 151
Critical, 165
Crocus, 50
Crotalus Cascavella, 72
Crotalus Horridus, 73, 74, 76
Croup, 119, 132, 231
Crowds
    fear of, 46, 183
    love of, 72
Cruelty, 21
Cults
    leaders, 208
Cunning, 234
Cuprum Metallicum, 77, 215, 244
Curare, 224, 245

Index

Curry, 111
Cyanosis, 85
Cystitis, 29, 34, 104, 182, 183
Cysts
 ovarian, 103

D

Dairy products
 averse to, 231
Damp, 24
Dancing
 loves, 79
 manic, 233
Dandruff, 92, 95
Dangle
 lets the affected part, 70
Dark
 fear of, 49, 148, 229
Day-blindness, 118
Dazed, 160
Deaf, 230
 sudden, 170
Death
 delusion of, 38
 delusion of, 74, 131
 dreams of, 74
 fear of, 46, 85
 feels close to, 203
 talks about, dispationnately, 245
 thinks of, when alone, 72
Decay, 100

Deceitful, 45
Deception, 218
Dehydration, 57, 118, 206
 diarrhoea, from, 238
Delicate, 62
Delirium, 89
Delusions, 18, 167
 air filled with perfume, 27
 animals, of, 167
 being in two different places, 52
 being singled out for divine vengeance, 130
 body is transparent, 27
 death, 38, 131
 dogs, sees, 167
 family, the, 131
 friends, has no, 172
 great person, of being, 167
 harassed, of being, 59
 has been abused, betrayed, 163
 injured, of being, 167
 insulted, of being, 167
 lawsuit, engaged in, 193
 madness, 52
 sex, 131
 they will lose their place in society, 240
 thinks he is a dog, 164
Dengue fever, 58
Denial, 218
Dental amalgam, 120

254

Index

Dependent, 161
Depravity, 44
Depression, 17, 64, 82, 91, 98, 108, 132, 154, 180, 183, 190, 220, 229
Deprivation, 71
Dermatitis, 95, 215
Despair, 142
Despondent, 85, 172
Destructive, 209
Detached, 51
Devil makes work for idle hands the, 132
Devoted, 145
Diabetes, 127, 206, 221
Diarrhoea, 29, 88, 173, 206, 237
  alternating with constipation, 104
  pains, abdominal, with, 238
Diesthylstilbestrol (D.E.S.), 104
Digestion, 128, 137, 146
  severe disorders, 237
Digitalis, 94
Dignified, 18
Dignity, 12
Dioscorea Villosa, 79
Dirty old man, 101
Discharges
  acid, 13
  acrid, 141
  black, 97

foul, 141
  lack of, when ill, 244
  opaque, 145
  suppressed, 220
  ulcerated, 13
Disciplined, 22
Disease
  fear of, 148
Disgust, 142
Disobedient, 13
Dissatisfied, 219
Distance
  misjudges, 207
Distended, 185
Dizziness, 66
Dog's milk, 147
Dogmatic, 55
Dogs
  fear of, 59, 149, 229
  love of, 149
Domineering, 87
Down's syndrome, 45
Drained, 105, 205
Dramatic, 244
Draughts
  aggravated by, 138
  sensitive to, 119
Drawn, 168
Dream
  as if in a, 117, 198
  in a, 50
Dreams
  business, 47
  dead, of the, 174

Index

fire,of, 167
  journeys, 47
  lost, in own house, 168
  lost, of being, 174
  never, 170
  robbers, of, 174
  violent, 52
  vivid, 27, 52, 159
Dress
  inappropriate, 70
Dressing up
  loves, 79
Drink
  alcohol, 163
Drinks
  warm, 167
Drosera, 164
Drowning
  fear of, 38
Drowsy, 27, 133
Drugs, 67, 177
  abuse of, 117
  history of taking, 199
  ill effects of, 51
Duality
  sense of, 203
Dulcamara, 87
Dull, 45
Dupuytren's contracture, 215
Duty, 130, 147
Dynasty, 208
Dysentery, 55, 146
Dysentery Co., 90, 110

Dysmenorrhoea, 63, 81, 104, 160
Dyspnoea, 86

E

Eager to please, 108
Ear, 175
Ears
  blocked, 145
Ears, 27
  discharge, 109
  scurf, 123
Eating, 24
  constant, 125
  refuses to eat, 236
Ebola virus, 39
Eccentric, 135
Ecstasy, 177
Eczema, 179, 202
  suppression of, 243
Edema, 53, 85, 118, 136, 186, 211, 221
  lungs, 15
Eggs, 108
  averse to, 231
Egocentric, 75, 207
Ejaculation, 164
  premature, 69
Elaps, 97, 163, 187
Electric Shock Treatment, 117
Emaciated, 32, 108, 125, 168, 213
Embittered, 193

Index

Emotions
   suppressed, 169
Emperor's new clothes, the, 209
Emphysema, 15
Endometriosis, 104, 174, 239
Energetic, 110, 233
Entrepreneurs, 136
Enuresis, 29, 244
Epilepsy, 44, 63, 116, 131, 200, 211, 230, 244
Eructations, 30, 94, 185
Eruptions, 95, 143
   pus, 166
   thick, hard, 202
Erythema, 182
Escape
   desire to, 198
Estrogen, 102
Eustachian tube, 122
Evil
   fear of, 49
Exaggeration, 49
Excitable, 108, 202
Exhausted, 62, 99, 229
Exhaustion, 79, 194, 205, 227, 242
Exhibitionists, 78
Exophthalmos, 126
Explosive, 193, 211, 244
Expression
   difficult, 166

Extrovert, 99
Eyelids
   cysts, 184
   red, sticky, 34
Eyes, 34, 88, 128, 170, 180, 184, 224, 226
   bags, 135
   black spots, 170
   blue, 108
   heavy lidded, 27
   puffy around, 135
   short-sighted, 75
   suppuration, 122

F

Face
   pains, nerves, 170
Faint
   feeling, before eating, 217
Fainting
   fear of, 148
Fair, 108
Fairground rides
   aggravated by, 32
Faithful, 149
Falling
   dreams of, 59, 85
   fear of, 97, 148
Family
   believes he was born into wrong, 209
Fanatical, 68, 165
Fastidious, 83
Fat

Index

averse to, 123, 231
craves, 195
unable to digest, 109
upset by, 231
Father, 12
Fatigue, 83
Fault-finding, 135
Fear, 161, 211
Fearful, 74, 85, 108, 230
Fearless, 199
Fears
  anticipatory, 90
Feet
  hot, 129
  one cold, other hot, 86
  soles dry, hot, wrinkled, 222
  sticks out of bed, 223
  sweaty, 185
Female organs, 17
Ferocious, 121
Ferrum, 177, 232, 243
Fever, 64
Fibrillation
  atrial, 86
  ventricular, 86
Fibroids, 103
Fibrositis, 93, 109, 181, 214, 231
Fibrous tissue, 224
Fidgety, 31, 64
Fields, W.C., 228
Fiery, 126
Figworts, 123

Fingertips
  icy, 154
Fire, 226
  dreams of, 84, 174
Fish, 109
  bone, sensation of, 120
Fissures, 143
  anal, 143
Flabby, 109, 229
Flatulence, 60, 137, 183, 191, 215
Flatus, 94
Floating
  felling of, 153
Flowers
  sensitive to smell of, 223
Fluid
  loss of, 57, 83
Fluoric Acid, 99, 140
Fluorine, 99, 125
Flying
  aggravated by, 32
  delusion of, 69
Folliculinum, 102, 103
Food
  fat, horror of, 145
Food
  assimilation, poor, 168
  aversion to, 89
  poisoning, 113, 238
Foolish, 239
Forgetful, 49, 52, 82, 149
Forsaken, 154, 162, 168, 240

Index

Frantic, 234
Fraxinus Americanus, 158
Freckles, 81
Freedom, desires, 101
Friendly, 242
Fright, fight, flight, 211
Frivolous, 188
Frolic
   desire to, 98
Fruit
   craves, 169, 206
Frustration, 55
Fun, 79
Future
   fear of, 91

G

Gaertner, 108, 229
Gallbladder, 59, 179, 191, 203, 222
Galley slaves, 97
Gallstones, 181, 192, 220
Gangrene, 39
Gas
   post-operative, 60
Gastric flu, 60
Gastric problems, 203
Gelsemium, 82, 224, 245
Genitals, 196
   sensitive, 166, 235
Gesticulating, 239
Ghosts
   fear of, 217

sees, 72, 89
Giggles, 49
Ginger, 112
Gingivitis, 93
Glands, 141
   indurated, 126
   swollen, 119, 150, 166
Glandular fever, 107
Glauber's Salt, 190
Glaucoma, 220, 226
Glonoine, 60
Gloomy, 59
Glossy magazines, 100
Glue ear, 146
Gold
   wears, 138
Gonorrhoea, 48, 112, 124
   suppressed, 191
Goose
   delusion, thinks he is a, 68
Gourmets, 80
Gout, 28
Grandeur
   delusions of, 50, 240
Graphites, 47, 96, 179, 202
Grass
   cut, 88
   desire to play in, 98
Grief, 11, 17, 71, 78, 162, 205
   ailments from, 127
   difficult, 136
Groin
   swellings in, 166

Index

Growing pains, 95
Growling, 164
Grudge, 13
Guilt, 130, 148, 157, 242
   religious, 166
Gums
   bleeding, 14, 220
Gunpowder, 112
Gunshot wounds, 112
Gymnasium
   visits daily, 234

H

Haemophilia, 39, 54, 73, 74
Haemorrhage, 39, 57, 74, 146
Haemorrhoids, 215
Hair
   brittle, 95
   thick, matted, oily, 167
Halliwell, Geri, 210
Hallucinations, 26
Hallucinogens, 177
Hamstrings, 19
Hands
   clammy, cold, 108
   one cold, other hot, 86
   wrings, 45, 131
Hangover, 160
Harsh, 12
Hateful, 21
Hatred, 12, 193
Haughty, 87, 142, 207

Hawking, Stephen, 82
Hay fever, 88, 92, 222
Head
   feels light, 167
   injury to, 116
   injury, mental troubles from, 190
   opening and closing, sensation of, 51
Headaches, 84, 92, 128, 160, 167, 179, 213, 216, 222, 237
   alternating, 150
   as if the skull would burst, 60
   chronic, 230
   light, from, 155
   menses, worse during, 230
   nail, like a, 224
   pressure, sensation of, 245
   sinus, from infection of, 230
Heart, 11, 21, 26, 28, 75, 85, 90, 124, 187, 224
   as if hanging by a thread, 137
   cardiovascular disease, 221
   fluttering, 94
   palpitations, 143
   right-sided symptoms, 158
   stitching pains around, 226
   valves, 187
Heartburn, 94, 181, 228
Heat, 103

Index

Hedonists, 99
Heights
   fear of, 32
Helleborus Niger, 114
Hemiopia, 230
Hemlock, 66
Hemp, 48
Hepar sulph, 119, 195
Hepatitis, 55
Heracleum Pirosella, 119
Herpes, 24, 88, 112, 124, 213
   zoster, 129
Hippies, 176
Hips
   pain, 109
Hoarders, 69, 138
Hoarseness, 123
Homesickness, 97, 205
Homœopathic lance
   the, 120
Hormone replacement therapy, 64, 80, 107
Horse riding
   ameliorates, 233
Hot flushes, 103
HRT, 64, 80, 107
Humiliation
   ailments from, 206
Hunger, 59
Hurried, 91, 99, 156, 227
Hydrophobia, 83, 161
Hydrophobinum, 161

Hyoscyamus, 77, 87, 161, 165
Hyperactive, 99, 109, 140, 227
Hyperactivity, 220, 234
Hyperglycaemia, 221
Hypersensitive, 102, 161
Hypersexual, 242
Hyperthyroidism, 93
Hypochondria, 195
Hypoglycaemia, 221
Hypothyroidism, 180
Hysterectomy, 70, 104
Hysteria, 72, 156, 173, 234

I

I.B.S., 221, 232
Ice
   craving for, 238
   sensation of, 238
Icy
   cold, 238
Idealistic, 13
Ideas
   has many, 58, 176
Identity
   doubts, 31
   loss of, 102, 105
Ignatia, 117, 166, 205, 212, 224
Imagination
   lacking, 190
Imbecility, 44

Index

Immune system
   depressed, 220
Impatient, 89, 91
Impetuous, 196
Impotence, 48, 69, 132
Incest, 131
Incoherent, 238
Indecisive, 64, 82, 103, 202
Independent, 38
Indian food, 111
Indifferent, 101, 114, 219
Indigestion, 94, 185
Induration, 68
Industrious, 233
Infection
   fear of, 46
Infections, 112
Infertility, 32, 159
Influenza, 231
Injuries slow to heal, 204
Inoculations
   horror of, 224
Insanity, 142, 239
   fear of, 64, 149
Insect bites, 113
Insecure, 90, 194
Insensitive, 44
Insomnia, 27, 95, 182
Intelligent, 38, 108
Intense, 163
Intestines, 15
Intoxication, 27
Intuitive, 79

Intussusception, 199
Iodum, 125, 165
Ipecac, 57
Irascible, 83
Iris Versicolor, 127, 128
Iritis, 181
Irresolution, 186
Irresponsible, 140, 176
Irritable, 59, 75, 108, 121,
   141, 142, 157, 159,
   168, 180, 183, 202,
   216, 219, 229, 243
   children, 170
Irritable bowel syndrome, 221,
   232
Irritated, 52, 230
Isolated, 114, 207
Isolation
   fear of, 72
Itching, 89, 143, 200
   urticarial, 110
Itchy bottom, 95

J

Jaundice, 76, 85, 181
Jaundiced, 168
Jealousy, 52, 72, 183
Jerking, 65, 200
Jesus, 50
Jewish humour, 138
Joints, 13
   swollen, 29
Joker, the, 239

Index

Junk food, 109
Justice
  desires, 80

K

Kali Arsenicum, 90
Kali Bichromium, 141
Kali Bromatum, 130
Kali Carbonicum, 53, 134
Kali Muriaticum, 109, 124, 145, 212
Kali Phosphoricum, 111
Kelp, 126
Ketosis, 109
Kidneys, 11, 28, 48, 124, 136, 146, 183, 211
  support, 30
Kill, desire to, 121, 200
Kleptomania, 83, 174
Knees
  pain, 19
Kundalini, 186

L

Labour, 63
  delusions of being in, 240
  pains, 35
Lac Caninum, 147, 164, 208
Lac Defloratum, 147, 154
Lac Humanum, 106
Lachesis, 11, 14, 53, 63, 73, 74, 77, 103, 141, 152, 186, 245

Lactose
  intolerant of, 154
Laryngitis, 175
Larynx, 175
  burning, 222
  suffocation, feeling of, 187
Lascivious, 240
Laudanum, 198
Laughter, 49
Lazy, 26
Lead poisoning, 201
Leather
  black, 54
Ledum, 167
Left side
  worse lying on, 189
Legs
  cramp, 146
  swollen, 39
Lemonade
  desires, 205
  likes, 197
Lethargic, 56
Leucorrhoea, 50, 109, 196, 232
Liars, 219
Libido
  high, 152, 156, 207
Light
  aversion to, 71
Lightning
  fear of, 74
Lilium Tigrum, 156, 188, 210
Lips

Index

cracked, 123
dry, cracked, 180
Listless, 15
Lively, 99, 140
Liver, 11, 30, 55, 59, 85, 123, 128, 171, 179, 191, 203, 222
   ailments in children, 172
Liverish, 183
Lobelia, 85
Lonely, 173
Loners, 212
Loquacious, 51, 63, 72, 74, 79, 126, 140, 239
Loss
   fear, pain of, 171
Lost, 97
Love, 12
   ailments from disappointed, 117
   cannot assimilate, 169
   first, 159, 206
Loyal, 147
LSD, 177
Lumbago, 181
Luna, 106
Lungs, 13
   oedema, 15
Lustful, 78
Lycopodium, 22, 36, 55, 57, 94, 97, 100, 118, 172, 179, 183, 230
Lying
   feels better by, 175
Lymph glands, 229
Lyssin, 161

M

M.E., 106, 220
Madness
   delusion of, 52
   fear of, 49, 64
   thinks is going mad, 165
Madonna, 210
Magnesia Carbonica, 79, 168
Magnesium Muriaticum, 172, 212
Magnesium Phosphoricum, 63
Malaria, 55, 58
Malicious, 142
Malnourishment, 108
Malnutrition, 221
Manganum, 175
Manic, 161, 163
Manic depressive, 174
Manipulative, 162
Marathon runners, 234
Marriage
   arranged, 65
Massage
   ameliorates, 233
Mastoiditis, 123
Masturbation, 44
Materialistic, 68
Maternal
   instinct lacking, 177

Index

Measles, 230
Meat, 19, 109
  craves, 169
Medorrhinum, 33, 48, 68, 99, 104, 157, 229
Memory, 23
  lacking, 115
Menière's disease, 214
Meninges
  irritation of, 230
Meningitis, 118, 191, 214, 230
Menopause, 63, 71, 73, 76, 103, 179, 243
Menses, 102, 103, 170, 211
  amelioration during, 245
  at night, 170
  convulsions around, 131
  extreme pain, 237
  heavy, 151
  irregular, 159
  pain, only when no, 170
  painful, 239
  profuse, 104
  red, dark spots, 104
  sleep, only during, 170
  sore throat at, 151
  sore throat before, 170
  weak, pale, 220
Menstruation, 103
  dark, 13
  Diarrhoea, vomiting, 20
  quarrelsome during, 16

Mercury, 110, 120, 165, 166, 195, 203, 228
Mescaline, 26
Miasms
  syphilitic, 110
  tubercular, 110
Mice
  delusions of, 64
Migraine, 76, 104, 128, 213, 223, 239
Milk, 29, 71, 108
  aggravates, 197
  allergic to, 173
  aversion to, 155
  breast, dries up, 151
  breast, promotion of, 151, 154
  sour, smells like, 169
  worse for, 34
Mind-body split, 22
Mirrors
  fear of, 47
Miscarriage, 50, 63, 156
Mischievous, 79, 83
Misfortune
  fear of, 46
Misleading, 78
Moles, 81
Moody, 52, 103, 243
Moon
  affected by, 166
  new, convulsions around, 131
Moors murderers, the, 54

Index

Moral, 186
Morbid, 186
Morgan, 96, 178, 179
  Gaertner, 183
Mother, 12, 17
Motion
  downward, fear of, 31
  sickness, 203
  worse on first, 93
Motor neurone disease, 82, 245
Mouth, 145
  cracks in corners, 180, 214
  dry, hot, 34
Mucous membranes, 14, 17, 32, 119, 229
Mucus, 173
Murder
  delusion of, 74
  impulse to, 126
Muscles, 62
Musculature
  underdeveloped, 108
Music
  ameliorates, 233
  aversion to, 45
  love of, 38, 72
  sadness from, 85
Myalgic Encephalitis, 106, 220

N

Nails, 95
  bites, 108, 229
  biting, 184
Naja, 52, 97, 163, 165, 186
Napoleon, 50
Nappy rash, 33, 244
Narcosis, 198
Nasal septum
  destruction of, 144
Natrum Carbonicum, 18
Natrum Muriaticum, 17, 68, 88, 105, 116, 117, 125, 155, 172, 205, 212, 219
Natrum Phosphoricum, 111
Natrum Sulphuricum, 34, 55, 58, 80, 116, 190
Nausea, 20, 62, 66, 85, 128, 181, 191, 223
Neck
  cervical problems, 222
  nerve damage in, 224
Necrosis, 39
Necrotising fasciitis, 39
Needles
  fear of, 224
Neglected
  feels, 186
Nephritis, 48, 146
Nerves, 62, 224, 242
  nervous breakdown, 184
  nervous system, 171, 211

Index

Nervous, 31, 62, 90, 108, 147, 168, 180, 229
Neuralgia, 92, 174, 184, 216, 226
   trigeminal, 225
Neuritis, 95
Neurotic, 77
Night
   blindness, 118
   fear of, 46, 49
   nightwatching, 62, 194
   terrors, 133
   worse, 142
Nitricum Acidum, 193
Noble, 186
Noise, 103
   aggravates, 91
   sensitive to, 244
Nose, 14, 175
   burning, 222
   catarrhal, 34
   crusts in, 97
   dry, congested, 222
   nosebleeds, 92
   red, 34
NSU, 48
Numb, 116
Nurturing, 12, 17
Nutrition, 108
   lack of, 154
Nux Vomica, 36, 69, 83, 94, 99, 224
Nymphomania, 131

O

Oatmeal, 108
Obedient, 147
Obese, 126
Obesity, 14, 17, 179
Oblomov's syndrome, 176
Obsessive, 90, 166
Obstinate, 142, 195
Odours, 200
Oedema, 53, 85, 118, 136, 186, 211, 221
   lungs, 15
Oestrogen, 102
Onions
   upset by, 231
Oopharinum, 102
Open air
   desires, 235
Opium, 26, 116, 198, 222, 239
Orange
   aversion to, 81
Oranges
   upset by, 231
Order
   likes, 111
Orphan's Remedy, The, 168
Osteoporosis, 221
Otitis media, 122, 184
Otorrhoea, 92, 180, 230
Outrage
   feelings of, 78
Ovaries, 188

Index

polycystic, 103
Overindulgence, 68
Oversensitive, 168, 219
Ovulation, 103
Ozoena, 144

P

P.M.S., 104, 160, 220
Pain, 171
  aching, 28
  agonising, 224
  burning, 213
  burning, spasmodic, 174
  cutting, 95, 138
  dull, 28
  high threshold, 219
  in heart, 28
  lumbo-sacral, 231
  over-sensitive to, 121
  painless, 116, 198
  relief of, 222
  sharp, 138
  splinter-like, 120, 195
  stitching, 138
Painters, 58
Pale, 168
Palms
  burning, 157
  dry, hot, wrinkled, 222
Palpitations, 28, 90, 94, 106
Pancreas, 127, 128
Pancreatitis, 221
Panic attacks, 103

Papaver, 198, 222
Paralysis, 66, 82, 97, 114
Paranoia, 72
Paranoid, 163
Parkinson's disease, 245
Passiflora, 214
Peacemaker, the, 172, 212
Pear-shaped, 213
Penetration
  fear of, 52
Perception
  changed, 48
  distorted, 25
Periods, 102
Peristalsis
  lacking, 199, 238
Persecuted, 132
Persecution
  sense of, 38
Perspiration, 119, 203
  at night, 110
  on head, at night, 230
Pertussis, 79
Perverted, 52
Pessimistic, 172
Petroleum, 179, 202
Phlebitis, 181, 214
Phlegm, 173
Phosphoricum Acidum, 205
Phosphorus, 36, 74, 100,
  109, 110, 117, 125, 242
Photophobia, 155, 191, 230
Pickles, 19

Index

Piles, 185, 215
Pill
   the morning after, 104
Pineal gland, 159
Pins
   fear of, 52, 224
Pit Viper, 52
Platina, 50, 156, 207
Playful, 188
Pleurisy, 216, 231
Plug in part
   delusion of, 22
   sensation of, 123
Plumbum, 199
Plump, 62
Pneumonia, 15, 136
Poets, 58
Police, 138
   dreams of being pursued by, 132
Policemen, 80
Pollution
   ill effects of, 227
Polybowel, 35
Polyps, 46, 222
   nasal, 184
Pork, 74
   better for, 217
Pornographers, 52
Possessive, 70
Posture
   lying, 18
Potatoes, 19
Practical, 55

Practical jokers, 79
Preachers
   in streets, 241
Precious, 207
Precocious, 110
Pregnancy, 35
   fear during, 64
   nausea, 63
   phantom, 50
   vomiting in, 155
Pre-menstrual syndrome, 104, 160, 220
Pressure
   around body, dislikes, 30
   better for, 33
   unbearable, 121
Prestige
   fear of losing, 97
Priapism, 48
Priests, 67, 158
Princess Diana, 64
Principled, 138
Prisoners, 67
Prolapse, 156, 167
Promiscuous, 152
Prostate, 69, 243, 245
Prostitutes, 78
Prostration, 146
Protective, 147
Proteus, 90, 106, 211
Proud, 207
Pruritus, 89, 182, 185, 215

Index

Psoriasis, 35, 95, 129, 143, 179, 183
Psorinum, 80
Psychopaths, 54
Puberty, 130, 159
Pulsatilla, 34, 62, 78, 105, 108, 110, 141, 152, 160, 162, 186, 203, 208, 217
Pulsations
   localised, 20
Pulse
   slow, 85
Punks, 13
Pupils
   dilated, 27
Purple, 14, 189
Pus, 120
Put upon, 97
Pyorrhoea, 184
Pyromaniacs, 122

Q

Quarrelsome, 69, 87, 142, 202, 217, 219
Quercus, 228
Quick-thinking, 165
Quinine, 57

R

Rabies, 163
Radiotherapy, 110, 117
Radium Bromatum, 217

Rage, 77, 161, 200
Raging, 161
Rain
   fear of, 97, 187
   hates, 163
Ranunculus bulbosa, 216
Rash
   measles, varicella, like, 230
Rats
   fear of, 64
Rattlesnake, 74
Raw, 12
Raynaud's syndrome, 95, 106, 214, 239
Rectum, 146
   stinging, 20
Refugees, 205
Relationships
   destroy, desire to, 100
   difficulty with, 25
Religious, 38, 165
   groups, 133
Remorse, 161
Repentance, 163
Rescuer, 105
Resentful, 12, 14, 17, 19, 78, 193
Respect, 12
Respiration, 136, 183
Responsibility, 12, 141, 176, 186
Resting, 103

Index

Restless, 53, 72, 89, 91, 131, 164, 168, 169, 183, 229, 245
Revolutionary, 13
Rheumatism, 29, 62, 88, 93, 150, 181, 216
Rhinitis, 92, 222
Rhus Toxicodendron, 24, 71, 132, 216
Rhythm
   ameliorates, 233
Ribs
   intercostal neuralgia, 185
Ridiculous, 239
Righteousness
   sense of, 241
Rio Carnival, 72
Ritualistic behaviour, 165
Rocked
   worse for being, 33
Rolls
   from side to side, 236
Romance
   loves, 79
Romantic poets, 198
Rose cold, 223
Rushed, 156, 228
Ruta, 196

S

S.A.D., 117
Sabina, 50
Saccharinum, 218
Sad, 74
Sadness, 17, 63, 162, 169
Safety
   longs for, 164
Salivation, 146, 166
   excess, 123
   profuse, ropy, 129
Salt, 71, 125, 173
   allergic to, 173
   averse to, 231
   craves, 167
Sanguinaria, 222
Sarcodes, 159
Sarsparilla, 172
Scarlatina, 94
Scars, 228
   itching, 189
Schizophrenia, 25, 45, 165, 186
School
   behind at, 168
   difficulties at, 133
Sciatica, 19, 47, 93, 142, 150, 239
Scolding, 87
Scorpion, 194
Scrofulous, 119, 128
Scrotum
   oedema of, 85
Sea, 125
   aggravations from, 173
   aggravations from, 32
Seashore, 228

Index

Seaside, 88
Seasonal Affective Disorder, 117
Secretions
　acid, 18
　Albuminous, 18
Secretive, 219
Security
　lacks, 169
Selenium, 243
Self-aware, 174
Self-confidence
　lacks, 148
Self-conscious, 174
Self-denial, 68, 105
Self-disgust, 147
Self-image
　inappropriate, 70
　poor, 165
Self-indulgent, 78
Selfish, 78, 162
Self-judgement, 219
Self-mutilation
　desire to, 165
Self-pity, 17, 217
Self-protective, 18
Self-reproach, 147
Self-worth, 12, 31
Senile dementia, 116
Senility
　premature, 69
Sensitive, 59, 62, 108, 119, 153, 162, 174, 224
　touch, to least, 169

Sensuality
　lacking, 77
Separation
　difficulty with, 106
Sepia, 35, 63, 69, 80, 104, 156, 159, 167, 179
Sepsis, 46, 57, 112, 143
Sex, 164, 243
　delusions of, 131
　mania, 240
Sexuality, 46, 207
　disturbed, 52
　sexual abuse, 53
　sexual erethism, 235
　strong, 104
　suppressed, 67, 130, 164
Shingles, 129, 216
Shock, 11, 70, 159
Shocks
　feels throughout body, 47
Shy, 90, 229
Sighing, 63, 85, 166
Sight
　dim, 220
Silica, 36, 80, 100, 109, 110, 120, 129, 180
Sinuses, 13, 18, 122, 141, 184
Skin, 24, 95, 202
　cracked, bleeding, 47
　eruption, convulsions following, 80
　eruptions, 166, 243
　eruptions suppressed, 118

Index

itching, 179
mottled, 189
oily, 229
rashes, 107
sensitive, 119
tearing at, 166
Sleep, 76
  aggravations from, 53
  fear of going to, 52
  restless, 182
  talks in, 15
  unrefreshed after, 169
  wakes unrefreshed, 159
  worse after, 39
Sleeplessness, 242
Sleepwalking, 133, 242
Sleepy, 82
Slow, 26
Sluggish, 17, 27, 119, 179
Smell
  sense of, distorted, 25
Smiling
  excessive, 239
Smoke
  worse for, 228
Smoking
  ill-effects of, 48
  worse for, 33
Snakebite, 186
Snakes, 148
  fear of, 147, 187
  snake remedies, 38
Snoring, 199

Snow Rose, 114
Sociable, 72, 75, 140, 147
Solidago, 30, 124
Somnambulism, 133, 199
Sour, 168
  craves, 33
  desires, 19
Sourness, 228
Spartium, 86
Spasmodic, 77
Spasms, 166, 211
Speech
  impaired, 72
  rapid, 214
  soft, 111
Spices
  craves, 223, 236
  desires, 123
Spigelia, 84, 224
Spine, 233
Spiritual, 38
  groups, 78
Spondylitis, 93
Spongia, 119, 127
Spots, 174
Spring
  like a coiled, 164, 233
Stab
  desire to, 59
Stammering, 225
Staphylococci, 122
Staphysagria, 106, 157, 161, 213

Index

Steroids, 80
Stings, 113
  fear of, 52
Stomach, 33, 59, 168
  aches, 109
  butterflies in, 137
  fluttering, 94
Stomatitis, 145
Stones
  renal, 183
Stools, 15, 20
  bloody, 39
  bloody, with spasms, 166
  cheerful after, 190
  clay, like, 168
  foul, 33
  grey, 29
  irritable before, 33
  loose, 95
  pain, on passing, 195
  spluttering, 192
  spluttery, green, 168
  yellow, 95, 228
  yellow, loose, 192
  yellow, soft, 215
Stramonium, 47, 83, 87, 116, 161
Streaks
  red, 46
Streptococcus, 74
Stress, 211, 242
Stroke, 116, 124
Strong-willed, 87

Stubborn, 69
Stuck
  when indicated remedy gets, 124
Study
  unable to, 82
Stutter, 166
Styes, 92, 180, 184
Sudden movements, 235
Sugar, 14, 19, 104, 108, 218
  averse to, 231
Suicidal, 72, 91, 117, 165, 186, 190, 240
Sulphur, 36, 50, 80, 178, 179, 192
Sulphuricum Acidum, 145, 227
Sunstroke, 200
Superficial, 100, 227
Superstitious, 68
Support
  lacks, 169
Suppression, 80, 244
  history of, 148
  of self, 68
Suppuration, 120
Suspicious, 52, 74, 98, 148, 193
Swallowing
  difficult, 53
  empty, worse for, 150
Swearing, 21, 78

Index

Sweat, 119
  cold, 237
  suprression of, 243
Sycotic Co, 229
Sympathetic, 75
Symptoms
  violent, 237
Syphilinum, 165, 166
Syphilis, 112, 128

T

Tabacum, 69, 85
Tachycardia, 94
Taciturn, 169
Talk
  about them, worse for hearing people, 16
  indisposition to, 240
  to self, 138, 217
  worse for, 14
Talkative. *See* Loquacious
Tantrums, 212
Tarentula Hispania, 233
Tarentula Hispanica, 47, 99
Tartrazine, 109
Taste
  bitter, 30
Tea
  averse to, 231
Tearful, 91
Tears
  lacking, 17
Teasing, 79

Teenagers, 45, 206
Teeth, 224
  abscess, 123
  pains, nerves, 170
Temper
  outbursts of violent, 219
Tendons, 19, 24
Tense, 77, 91, 180, 183, 229
Testicles, 142
Theatrical, 157
Thin, 108, 125, 170, 213
Thirst, 118, 160
Thirstless, 118
Thoughts
  out of control, 126
  two trains of, at same time, 165
  vivid, 58
Threatened, 194
Throat, 141
  burning, 222
  clears constantly, 175
  dry, burning, 180
  dry, constricted, 187
  heat rising to, 30
  lump in, 30
  lump in, 93
  mucus in, 231
  raw, dry, 231
  red, dry, constricted, 38
  spasms of, 166
Thrombosis, 39

Index

Thrush, 34, 145, 220
Thuja, 34, 48, 64, 68, 80, 90, 106, 131, 191, 195, 229
Thunder
 fear of, 74, 153
Thyroid, 125, 141
Thyroidinum, 105
Tidy, 111
Tight, 24
 averse to t. clothing around waist, abdomen, 123
Time
 11 a.m., 181
 11 p.m., 33
 12 a.m. – 3 a.m., 119
 2 - 3 a.m., 95
 2 - 3 a.m., 128, 231
 3 - 4 a.m., 17
 3 – 6 a.m., 96
 3 a.m., 15
 4 – 8 p.m., 118, 183
 4 a.m., 56
 4 p.m., 56, 93
 5 – 8 p.m., 158
 9 – 10 a.m., 93
Timid, 18, 74
Tinnitus, 60, 142
Tired, 14, 175
TNT, 193
Toad, 44
Tobacco
 aversion, to smoke, 224
 much worse for, 226
Tongue
 cracks in, 220
 fissures, 230
 furry, 230
 spongy, 29
 swollen, 180
 ulcers, on tip, 93
Tonsillitis, 93, 122, 150, 184, 230
Tonsils
 overgrown, 230
 swollen, 113
Toothache, 170
Tormented, 161
Torturer, 22
Touch, 103
 aggravated by, 137
 aversion to, 142
 sensitive to, 225
 sensitive to least, 235
Tourette's syndrome, 78
Trance
 in a, 114
Trapped
 fear of being, 235
Trauma, 11
 aetiology of, 199
Travel sickness, 32, 111, 203
Trembling, 200, 228, 243
Tubercular adenitis, 119

Index

Tuberculinum, 68, 74, 90, 91, 126, 217, 229
Tumours, 46
Twitching
  from suppression of discharge, 243

U

Ulcers, 29, 39, 137, 221
  corneal, 122
  duodenal, 94, 211
  mouth, 214, 220, 227
  peptic, 25
  varicose, 181
Unconscious, 238
Undernourished, 170
Unfeeling, 21, 83, 142
Unforgiving, 193
Unknown
  fear of, 32
Unmotivated, 159
Unselfish, 172
Unsure, 102
Unworthy, 147
Urethra
  burning, 109
Urethritis, 48, 191
Urinary tract, 183
Urination
  after headache, 128
  desire, 166
  painful, 48
Urine, 15
  dribbling, 29
  red sediment, 189
  retention of, 200
  strong, 28, 196
Uterus, 46, 63, 188
  retroverted, 156

V

Vaccination, 76, 79, 113
  rabies, 163
Vagina
  discharge, 195
  dryness, 103
  vaginitis, 183
Varicella, 230
Vasectomy, 70
Vegetables
  craves, 169
Veins
  like cold water running through, 238
  varicose, 181
Venus, 77
Veratrum Album, 97, 165, 237
Verrucas, 123
Vertebrae, 62
Vertigo, 66, 84, 86, 91, 153, 155, 214
Vescicles, 24
Vexatious, 69
Vicious, 21, 83
Vinegar, 36

Index

Violent, 161
Vision
　disturbed, 129
Visions, 27
Vitality
　low, 13
Vivacious, 38, 73
Voices
　hears, 50, 187, 209
Vomiting, 66, 86, 109, 128, 181
　drinking, after, 33
　with headaches, 223

W

Wallowing, 186
Wander
　desire to, 91
Warts, 88, 95, 124, 195, 229
　anal, 232
　flat, 182
Washing
　averse, 13
Water
　ailments from excessive, 191
　contaminated, 112
　dislikes, 228
　fear of, 38, 161
　running, 166
　trickling, sensation of, 51
Water brash, 94

Weak, 13, 143, 170, 227
　intellectually, 44
Weather
　aggravated by stormy, 216
　cold, damp aggravates, 89
　hot, worse in, 129
　wet, worse in, 191
Weepy, 74, 103, 180, 229
Weight, 103
　gain, 179
Wet-nurses, 149
Wheat, 104
Wheezing, 231
Whooping cough, 79
Widows, 67
Wild-looking, 163
Willpower, 26
Wind
　as though blowing on a part, 121
Wine, 29, 36
　aggravated by, 215
　easily drunk on, 246
Wires
　encaged in, delusion, 65
Withdrawn, 18, 116, 169, 172
Wolf spider, 233
Words
　forgets, 39
Work
　dislikes, 58
　fear of, 217
Worms, 110, 113, 225

Index

Wounds
  blue, 166
  difficult to heal, 112
  heal too quickly, 163, 166
  inflamed, 166
Wronged
  delusions of being, 156
  feeling of being, 163

Y

Yawning, 200
Yellow, 76, 92
Yielding, 80
Yoghurt, 191
Yogic mystics, 115

Z

Zincum, 80, 106, 242
Zingiber, 112